EXILES IN NEW YORK CITY

EXILES IN NEW YORK CITY

WAREHOUSING THE MARGINALIZED ON WARD'S ISLAND

PHILIP T. YANOS

Columbia University Press
New York

Columbia University Press
Publishers Since 1893
New York   Chichester, West Sussex

Copyright © 2025 Columbia University Press
All rights reserved

Cataloging-in-Publication Data available from the Library of Congress.

ISBN 9780231212366 (hardback)
ISBN 9780231212373 (trade paperback)
ISBN 9780231559348 (ebook)

LCCN 2024048100

Cover design: Julia Kushnirsky
Cover image: New Kirby Forensic Psychiatric Center at the Manhattan Psychiatric Center on Ward's Island, New York.
Courtesy of STV (photographer: David Cooper)

FOR ALL THOSE LIVING
BEHIND THE FENCES

CONTENTS

Acknowledgments ix

1 A STRANGE JUXTAPOSITION
1

2 WARD'S ISLAND:
A PLACE WHERE NO ONE WOULD COMPLAIN
18

3 PARKLAND OR INSTITUTIONAL
DUMPING GROUND?
38

4 THE *FRENCH CONNECTION* CONNECTION
54

5 "IN ACCORDANCE WITH THE STANDARDS"
71

6 WHERE WILL THESE CHILDREN PLAY?
87

7 "WE ARE NEW YORK'S FORGOTTEN PEOPLE":
THE ISLAND NOW
101

8 THE FUTURE: WHAT CAN WARD'S ISLAND BECOME?
118

Notes 139
Index 165

ACKNOWLEDGMENTS

Many people have made it possible for me to write this book. First, I must thank my family of origin—my mother, father, and brother—who shared the experience of living on Ward's Island with me during the 1970s. Although my father passed away several years ago, his photo collection, along with the many stories he told me over the years, made an important contribution to the book. My mother and brother both helped by sharing photos and memories and giving me permission to publish them. We all experienced living on Ward's Island together—I love you, and thank you so much for your support with this project!

This book would also not have been possible without the contributions of students working with me on my research team at John Jay College (the Mental Health Recovery Research Lab). Sheharyar Hussain and Melissa Martinez have been particular advocates, participating in several of the research studies and reading early drafts of chapters. Thank you so much for believing in this project! Other lab members who conducted research interviews and/or analyzed data include Samin Ali, Francesca Bellisario, Wen Ying Chen, Anna Mundy, Maria Muniz-Hernandez, Emma Nolasco, Beatrice Quijada, Lotus Schuller, and Ashley Sedlazek. I thank all of you for devoting your time and energy to assisting me with the research discussed in the book and for believing in its value.

I also thank the colleagues whom I interviewed for this book, including several who participated in confidential interviews, as well as Paul Piwko, founder and codeveloper of the National Museum of Mental Health Project, and Lisa Green, chief program officer for residential services at the Bridge, Inc. Thank you also to Dr. Gabriel Koz and Pamela Koz for answering my phone call and for mailing me a copy of *Made in South Africa*. A special thanks to my former mentee (now professor) Jospeh DeLuca, who read and provided invaluable feedback on the book proposal. I also thank the many professionals who informally shared their thoughts about the idea for this book, both while I was preparing it and after my presentation at the 2023 ISPS-US conference. I am especially grateful to Nev Jones and Jessica Arenella for providing me with encouragement and feedback. Thank you all for sharing your time, expertise, and experiences with me and making this much a better book!

I want to thank the community of lived experience advocates who have encouraged me to pursue this project, including Dan Frey, Helen "Skip" Skipper at City Voices, and Jessie Roth and Sascha Dubrul at IDHA. You all inspire me to keep going through all the discouragement of working in a deeply flawed mental health service system.

I also thank all of the clients who have given me the privilege of working with them over the years, especially those whose journeys have brought them into contact with the institutions of Ward's Island. Thank you for sharing your experiences with me and for giving me the chance to try to assist you through difficult times. I think about you often.

I also thank Stephen Wesley at Columbia University Press for believing in this project from the get-go and for encouraging me throughout the process. Thank you to Kathryn Jorge, Alex Gupta, and Peggy Tropp, who have guided the book through the production process. The colleagues who anonymously reviewed the proposal as well as the first draft of the book also provided very helpful feedback. I know that reading book proposals and full books is a largely thankless effort—so I thank you for doing it!

I also want to thank the librarians at John Jay College, especially those in the interlibrary loan division, who helped me tremendously in acquiring source material for the book. I don't know the names of everyone who helped, but I thank you. I especially want to thank Dr. Kathleen Collins, whose efforts to help me obtain an elusive source document were nothing short of heroic! Thank you to librarians at the Graduate Center who also assisted me directly, including Roxanne Shirazi, Awilda Ojeda, and Curtis Matthew. I really appreciate the time you took to assist me. Thank you also to the librarians at the New York Public Library, New York City Municipal Archives, New-York Historical Society, and New York Academy of Medicine, whose names I don't know. Your professionalism and dedication are inspiring.

Last, I must thank my family: my partner, Victoria Frye, and my children, Theo and Lexy. Tory, you are my love—thank you so much for your unwavering support throughout this process and your belief in it and me! I couldn't have (and wouldn't have) stuck with it without your love and support. Lexy, thanks for hanging in there with all of my stories of my childhood on Ward's Island, for walking with me through the island from the Bronx, and for all of your hugs. I want to finally and especially thank my son Theo, an aspiring urban planner, who helped tremendously by guiding me toward resources within the urban planning field, reading full drafts of the entire book and provided feedback on them, and even helping me get hold of an important source book that was available through his institution's library (but not mine). You rule! I hope I will be able to return the favor on a book that you write someday. Love you.

EXILES IN NEW YORK CITY

1

A STRANGE JUXTAPOSITION

In the summer of 2013 I had been working with Carlos as a psychotherapist for almost a year, and things had never been quite right for him during that time period.[1] Carlos, diagnosed with schizophrenia in his early twenties, hospitalized several times, and homeless for a stretch, was now in his late forties and had been living stably in the community for roughly fifteen years, residing in an apartment and staying out of the hospital for a lengthy period. He was a good-natured and likable person, seen as a model client in some respects by the agency that provided him with mental health services, with which I worked as a part-time provider. However, when I was asked to start working with him, things were not going so well. Carlos had become increasingly hostile toward team members, and they were concerned that he was heading for a major recurrence of the psychotic symptoms he had not experienced for a long time. I was asked to work with Carlos because we had good rapport from years of seeing each other around the clinic, and he seemed to trust and respect me, so the team was hoping I could help him get back to his baseline. Although we came from different backgrounds (I from a considerably more privileged one), we had some things in common: we were both native New Yorkers, were around the same age, and could connect on what things were like "back in the day" in our hometown.

2 A STRANGE JUXTAPOSITION

Despite this connection, when I met with Carlos, he seemed distant and less trusting. Gone were the sense of humor and easy conversation I had known, and despite our rapport and mutual positive regard, we struggled to develop a therapeutic alliance around what goals to work on together. It appeared to all that Carlos's psychotic symptoms, especially suspiciousness and a belief that he was being monitored by his neighbors and the police, were returning, despite evidence that he had been taking antipsychotic medication regularly as prescribed. This led to a series of short-term hospitalizations at city-run hospitals. Many times that I was scheduled to meet with Carlos for therapy ended up being replaced by visits to hospital units where he had been involuntarily admitted. At one of them, the hospital team stated that he was not improving and recommended that he be transferred to a state hospital, where he could be given more time to improve in response to a new medication. This was an outcome I had dreaded, because I worried that entering a state hospital, where stays could last more than six months, would jeopardize both his housing and his connection to the treatment team I worked with, which had been such important parts of his long stretch of community stability. Both housing and community-based treatment were at risk because while he was living in a state hospital his supplemental security income (SSI) would be discontinued, meaning he would be unable to pay his portion of his apartment's rent, and because the treatment team rules required that a client residing in a state hospital for more than three months be discharged from treatment.[2]

In the late summer of 2013, after returning from vacation, I was informed that what I feared had come to pass: Carlos had been transferred to the Manhattan Psychiatric Center, a state hospital located on Ward's Island, New York City. After roughly one month, we received word that Carlos was on a new medication, was doing a lot better, and would appreciate a visit from his community-based treatment team. I volunteered to visit, both because I cared about Carlos and wanted to support him and because I had a special interest in traveling to Ward's Island.

I was particularly interested in going to Ward's Island because I had essentially grown up there, living there for ten years, from 1970 to 1980, at roughly the ages of one to eleven. My family had moved there from our previous apartment in Queens to take advantage of an opportunity to live in a house (or "cottage") rented from New York State, my father's employer. My father, who had taken a job as a psychiatrist at what was then called Manhattan State Hospital, was apparently drawn in by the appeal of having a house within New York City, a yard where his young children could play, a very affordable rent (I remember being told that the initial rent was less than $100 per month, a great bargain even in 1970), and an extremely short commute to his job. Given that he had a car and liked to drive, the fact that the house was located on an island without amenities or reliable public transportation did not seem to have concerned him much, since he could easily drive to Manhattan. Ward's Island is near an off-ramp from the Triborough Bridge.

Ward's Island is nominally part of Manhattan's East Harlem neighborhood (in zip code 10035) and sits across the East River from an area running from approximately 99th to 115th Street (see figure 1.1).[3] It is connected by landfill to neighboring Randall's Island, which continues past 125th Street to the southern coast of the Bronx, where Manhattan Island begins to narrow. The Manhattan Psychiatric Center (previously Manhattan State Hospital) is one of five state-run psychiatric hospitals located within New York City's boundaries.[4] It consists of two imposing yellow brick buildings that are easily visible from the Harlem River Drive and its accompanying bike path in Manhattan (see figure 1.2). At one time Manhattan State Hospital was the largest psychiatric hospital in the United States, housing up to eight thousand adults,[5] but the Manhattan Psychiatric Center's current census capacity is limited to 240 and actually hovers around 150.[6] Although more than one hundred thousand cars drive over Ward's Island every day (according to state toll data) on the Triborough Bridge overpass that one might take if traveling from Manhattan to LaGuardia Airport,[7] most drivers and passengers have no idea what the island is or the nature of the lives of those who reside there.[8]

I elected to visit Carlos on a Friday in late August even though it was not one of the regular days on which I worked with the treatment team. I did this because I had extra time then, and I knew from previous experience that traveling to and from Ward's Island could take hours.

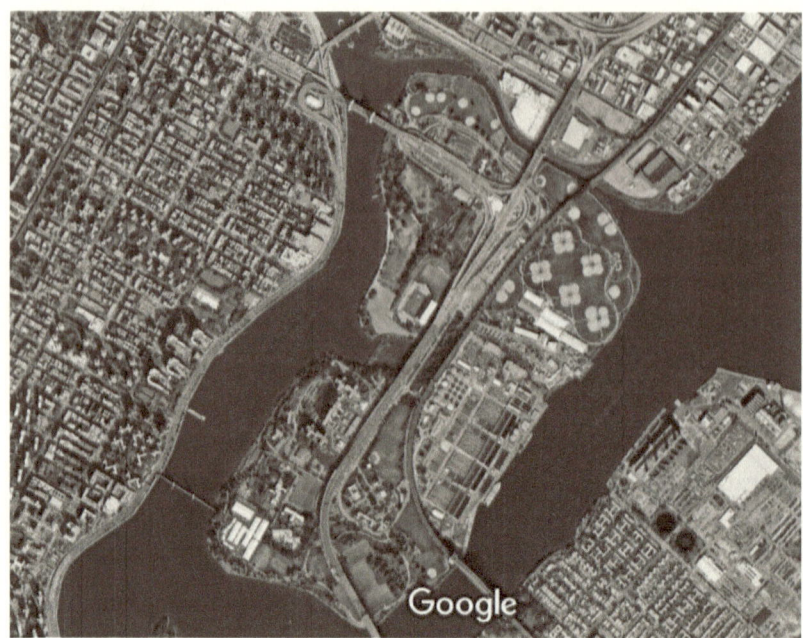

FIGURE 1.1 Aerial view of Ward's Island and Randall's Island, with East Harlem to the west, Queens to the east, and the Bronx to the north.

Source: Google Earth.

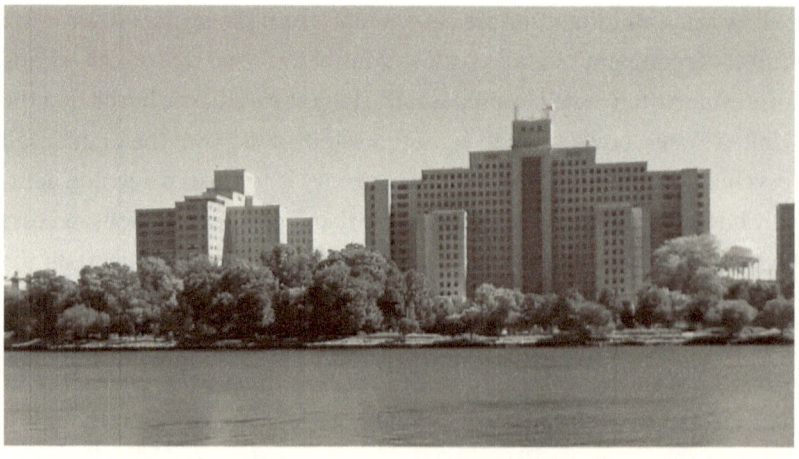

FIGURE 1.2 Manhattan Psychiatric Center on Ward's Island as seen from East Harlem, September 26, 2022.

Source: Photo by author.

Although the island is separated from Manhattan only by an approximately quarter-mile-wide stretch of water, it is accessible by public transportation only via a single bus line (the M35) that travels to and from a stop at the corner of 125th Street and Lexington Avenue in East Harlem. Although I had not taken it in years, I knew that the bus was infrequent and that I should therefore allow extra time. It had been more than twenty years since I had last been on the island, and I was filled with both nostalgia and curiosity as I walked across Manhattan on 125th Street. However, as I arrived at Lexington Avenue, I was caught by surprise and soon realized that there was something else going on that would make it considerably more difficult to reach the island. At the bus stop I saw not just the usual group of middle-aged adults associated with the island's various institutions, but scores of young people in their late teens and early twenties, most dressed as if going to the beach and with glitter on their faces. I then realized that today was one of the days on which the Electric Zoo Festival, an annual electronic music gathering attended by roughly a hundred thousand people, would be taking place on Randall's Island at a concert and sports pavilion that had been developed there, called Icahn Stadium.

I quickly reconfigured my plans and decided instead to walk on the pedestrian path of the Triborough Bridge (also known as the Robert F. Kennedy Bridge). Although I knew that the bridge and its overpass would travel over Ward's Island and continue on to Queens, I was fairly certain there was a ramp I would be able to take to walk down to Ward's Island. As my walk progressed over Randall's Island, I could hear the insistent beat of electronic music and see the tens of thousands of enthusiastic revelers dancing and cheering below. Ahead lay the institutions of Ward's Island: the Manhattan Psychiatric Center, where I was going; the Kirby Forensic Psychiatric Center, a related state institution for people who have been charged with a crime but deemed not competent to stand trial; the large Keener and Clarke Thomas Men's Shelters; two community residences for former hospital residents; and a residential substance use treatment program managed by Odyssey House. How strange it must be for the residents, I thought, to hear this music and see all of this revelry as they endure what is probably a very difficult period in their lives. Being on the island always gave a sense of being close to, but apart from, the opportunities and challenges of New York City, but this was bringing the city even closer to home, as there was no way one could not hear the music from this open-air festival. As I continued to walk, I found that there was indeed a ramp that I could take down to Randall's Island, where I could then walk over the roadway connection to Ward's Island and the entrance to Manhattan Psychiatric Center. As I entered Ward's Island, I could see that the area where the house that I had grown up in had been was now a grassy expanse surrounded by a fence (see figures 1.3 and 1.4). There appeared to be uniformed teenagers playing sports there. This was because of an arrangement between New York City and a federation of private schools (the Private School Athletic Association) to use public land on Ward's Island for their sports programs, something that I had heard about but was still taken aback to see.[9]

Finally, I reached the Manhattan Psychiatric Center and, after gaining access to the grounds by showing ID, I decided to take a short walk around the campus. However, I could see that the wooded area leading to the shoreline, where my brother and I would sometimes sit and skip rocks in the water while looking at Manhattan, was no longer accessible from the hospital grounds (see figure 1.5). There was now an attractive bike path on the shoreline, but instead of being accessible, it was separated from the hospital grounds by a high fence (see figures 1.6 and 1.7). This struck me as cruel. What was the purpose of this fence? To keep the hospital and other island residents from being able to access a public park space where they might interact with people deemed more worthy of enjoying it? Who had a greater right to it than *they*, those who actually lived on this island, for whom access to natural beauty might provide some refuge from the turbulence of their lives? What kind of message of exclusion did this convey to those residents? I was filled with outrage as I circled back to try to gain access to the inside of the Manhattan Psychiatric Center.

The last time I had been inside the hospital was in the early 1990s (roughly ten years after my family moved off the island), when I worked there as a volunteer, an experience that ended up being formative in my

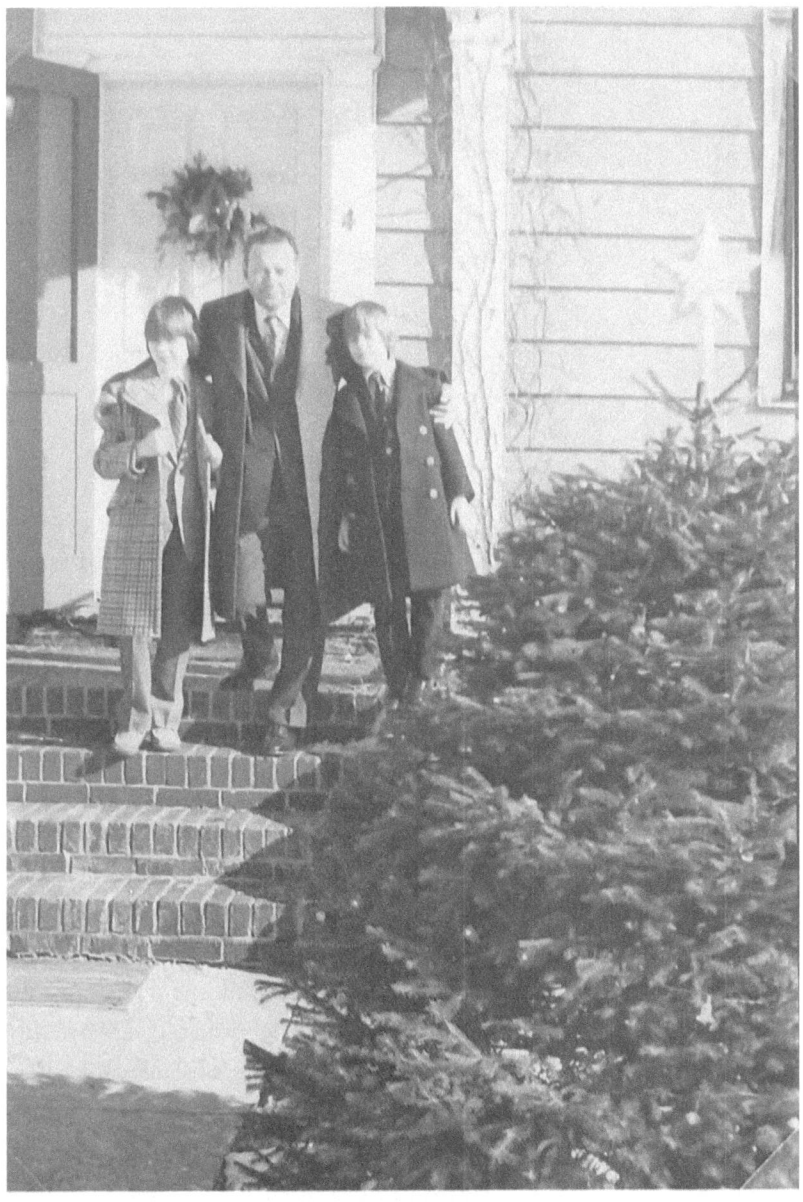

FIGURE 1.3 The author (*right*) with his father and brother in front of "Cottage 4," 1970s.

Source: Photo by Theodore Yanos.

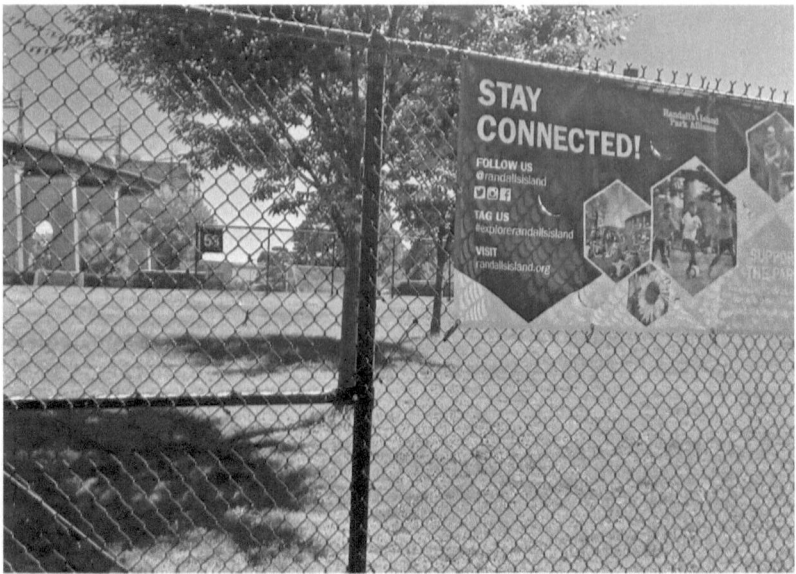

FIGURE 1.4 Sports field used by the Private School Athletic Association, September 26, 2022.

Source: Photo by author.

decision to pursue a career in clinical psychology focusing on people diagnosed with schizophrenia and other forms of psychosis. At that time, entering the hospital was not a complicated affair: you just walked in, maybe flashed an ID, but might not even need to do that. You could easily cross over from the Meyer to the Dunlap building using the connecting passage, then take the elevator up to the unit you were heading for and ring the doorbell. Units were locked, but someone would open the door for you and let you in with just a little explanation. Today it was different. Security would only admit me into the building after a call to the unit staff member I had spoken to in advance about my visit. I had to surrender my cell phone prior to entry. I had to pass through a section where one heavy door would close before another could open. This was much more like a jail than a hospital.

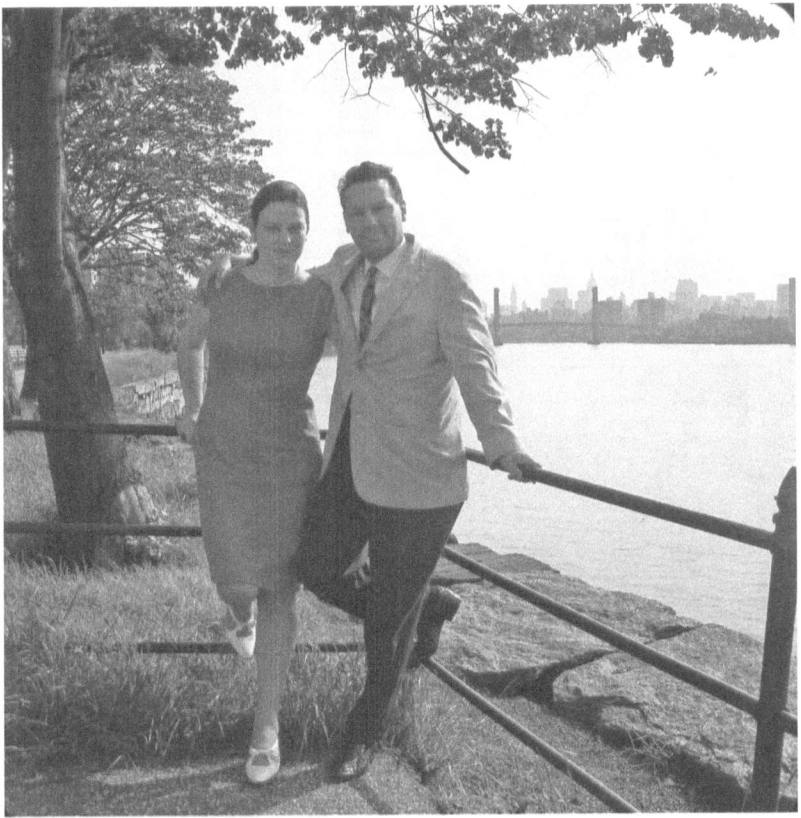

FIGURE 1.5 The author's parents on the Ward's Island shoreline in 1967.

Source: Photo by Theodore Yanos.

When I finally arrived on the unit, I was allowed to meet with Carlos, and he was very appreciative of my visit. Outside, I could still hear the bass drum thumping of the Electric Zoo, but it did not seem to register for Carlos. I found him to be much more like his old self than when I had last seen him—lucid, thoughtful, with a sense of humor, somewhat embarrassed that his symptoms had returned, but also confused because he had never stopped taking prescribed medication or relapsed on street drugs (a major factor in his initial development of psychosis as a young man). This led us to talk about the unfairness of

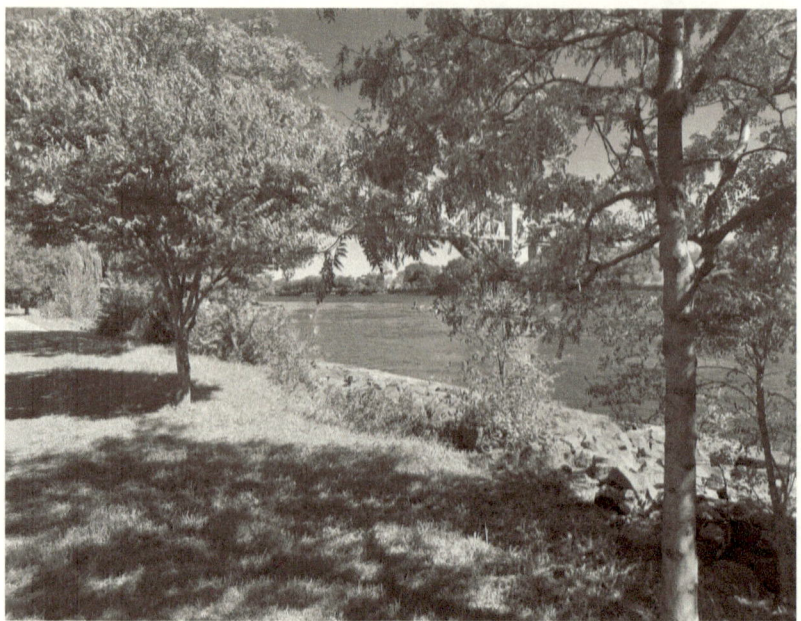

FIGURE 1.6 Ward's Island's shoreline and bike path, September 26, 2022.

Source: Photo by author.

psychosis and some of the circumstances that might have contributed to his recent psychiatric relapse. Carlos talked about how his apartment building in Manhattan was becoming increasingly gentrified and how he felt that residents were increasingly paying negative attention to him rather than ignoring him as they had for so many years. He started to suspect that they were spying on him, trying to get him kicked out, and maybe calling the police on him. Carlos, like many men of color growing up in New York City, had had several negative interactions with the police over the years and feared coming into conflict with them above all else.[10] He would often cross the street to avoid police officers if he saw them standing outside. As a young man experiencing psychosis for the first time, he had experienced use of force from the police while being taken to a psychiatric hospital for his first involuntary stays. Carlos's

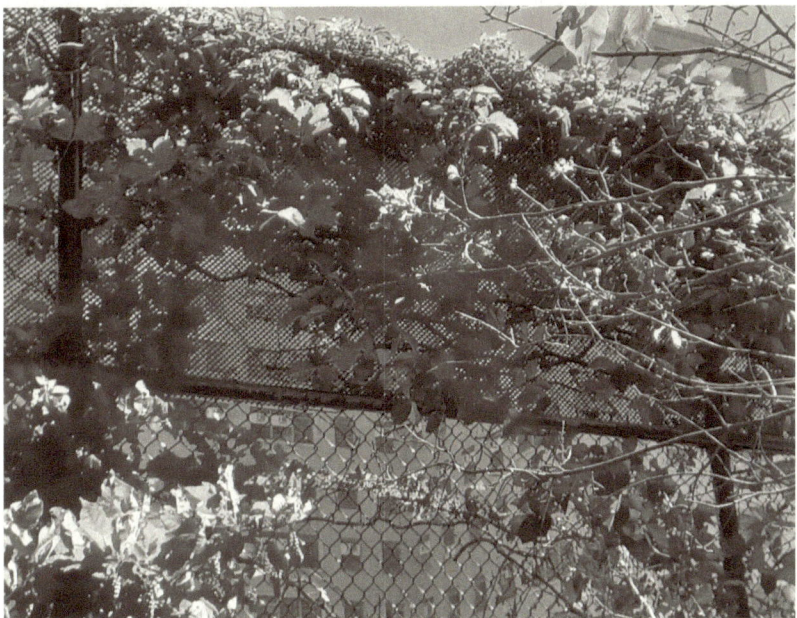

FIGURE 1.7 Fence separating Manhattan Psychiatric Center from shoreline, September 26, 2022.

Source: Photo by author.

feelings about gentrification were similarly sensitive and wrapped up in his personal story. He liked to say that he grew up in a "psychological borderland" in a poor racial and ethnic minority neighborhood in Manhattan that was close to a wealthy and predominantly white neighborhood. Although he could easily visit the wealthier neighborhood and take advantage of its many cultural institutions, he was nevertheless on the other side of a seemingly unsurmountable racial and economic divide. Following what is known as a cognitive behavioral therapy for psychosis approach,[11] Carlos and I talked about how there was plausibly an element of truth to the persecutory ideas he had developed—that his neighbors, recognizing him as someone who received mental health services, were watching him with suspicion. However, his psychosis had probably taken this reality and exaggerated it such that it became an overwhelming preoccupation that interfered with his sleep, further increasing his symptom severity. Carlos thought that this made sense and wished that he had seen it that way earlier.

At the end of my one-on-one meeting with Carlos, we met together with a staff member on the unit with whom he was working individually. The staff member agreed that Carlos was doing well but regrettably informed me that it would be several more months before he could be discharged. Once a person is admitted to the state hospital, there is a bureaucratic process of approval by a committee of psychiatrists that has to be followed in order for one to be discharged. Another issue was housing, since it was (and is) illegal for a state hospital to discharge someone to the streets or a shelter. As I had feared, Carlos's long stay in the hospital had led to his losing his longtime apartment in the community, and he could not be discharged until he had a new place to live. This was a lengthy process that could extend his inpatient stay for several more months. It might mean that he would have to live for some time in the Transitional Living Residence (TLR) also located on the island. The length of time this process would take meant that Carlos would be discharged from his community-based treatment team (which I worked with) since we had a limited caseload and, as a standard practice, discharged clients who were hospitalized for longer than three months. Carlos was sad, but understanding, about both of these realities and agreed that he should focus on the future and cementing his newly acquired psychiatric stability. I offered to visit him again in about a month, prior to his discharge from the team, and asked if it would be allowable for me to bring him a book to read that I thought might interest him. Carlos stated that he would love this, the team member approved it, and we agreed to meet again the following month.

When I returned, I found Carlos still doing well and hoping to be discharged soon. With permission from the treatment team, I offered him a book about the police corruption scandals in New York City in the 1970s, and he gladly accepted it. Carlos in turn gave me a card in which he thanked me for my dedication to helping him "through thick and thin" and stated that I was a "true humanitarian." I was sincerely moved by this and still keep the card. This was the last time I saw Carlos, who was transferred off the treatment team I worked with shortly after our meeting.

THE MEANING OF WARD'S ISLAND

Why does Ward's Island, what it was and has become, and what it means for the lives of people like Carlos—ordinary (and in many instances good) people who have experienced oppression in their lives and have fallen on hard times for one reason or another—matter to me, and why do I believe that it should matter to others? Ward's Island is a unique location within New York City in that, on any given day, it houses roughly 1,300 predominantly (roughly 85 percent) Black and Latino/a/x marginalized people in its two psychiatric hospitals, two homeless shelters, residential substance use treatment program, and two congregate housing facilities.[12] At the time of this writing, as discussed in chapter 7, the island is also the location for a two-thousand-bed shelter housing international migrants seeking asylum.

The majority of the island's residents have been diagnosed with a serious mental illness and/or have experienced substance use problems and are therefore in need of considerable support. Yet Ward's Island has no grocery stores, convenience stores, pharmacies, restaurants, coffee shops, libraries, banks, houses of worship, or any other amenities to offer its residents (a Protestant church that stood on the hospital grounds is now shuttered). There is only one public transportation source for getting on and off the island, the M35 bus (see figure 1.8), which is scheduled to travel every ten minutes during rush hour and every twenty minutes during off hours but is known to be considerably less reliable. It deposits passengers at the corner of 125th Street and Lexington Avenue, a location known as a nexus of drug commerce.[13] The island offers considerable green space for recreation, but, as previously noted, these areas have recently been separated by fence from the institutional facilities of the island, further isolating the island's residents from the rest of the city.

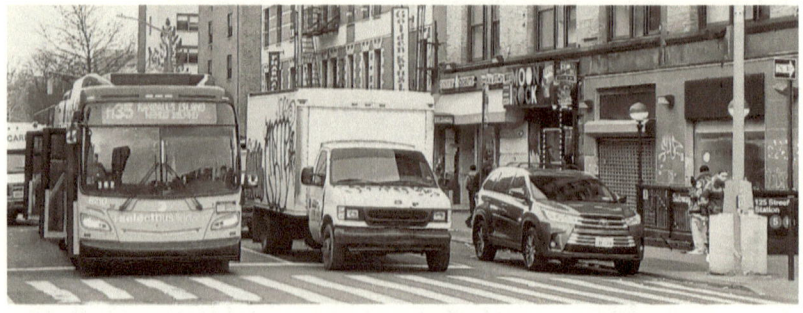

FIGURE 1.8 The M35 bus at 125th Street and Lexington Avenue in East Harlem, February 9, 2024.

Source: Photo by author.

Ward's Island's status as a location of urban exile is nothing new; it dates back almost 180 years, with the types of institutions that have been located on it remaining remarkably consistent. In the 1840s, it was selected as the location of the State Emigrant Refuge for "sick and destitute" immigrants (services that would later be provided on Ellis Island, in New York Harbor). There is evidence that the island also served as the location of several "potter's fields," or mass graves for poor New Yok City residents, burying tens of thousands of people during the mid-1800s. Soon thereafter, the island would accommodate an Inebriate Asylum (opened in 1868), for people with what would now be called alcohol use problems. Finally, the New York City Asylum for the Insane (the precursor to today's state psychiatric hospitals) was built and opened in the 1870s. The asylum, originally run by New York City and housing only men, converted to serving both sexes and grew in scope and size in the early twentieth century after its takeover by New York State.[14] Although Blackwell's Island (now Roosevelt Island), another island in the East River that was a prominent location for New York City public institutions in 1800s, is now completely free of them, Ward's Island's status as the location of multiple institutions for the social marginalized has persisted and in some ways continues to grow.[15]

The use of a remote urban area as a "dumping ground" for socially marginalized persons is certainly consistent with the way members of stigmatized groups have been treated over the past five hundred years, beginning with the development of "madhouses" in medieval England and France; for example, Paris's Hospital Bicetre, an early "madhouse" discussed at length by Michele Foucault in *Madness and Civilization*, was located on the far southern fringe of the city.[16] When asylums began to be built in the United States, it was recommended that they be located at least two miles away from urban areas.[17] Stigma theory predicts that one of the motivations for stigma toward people with certain marginalized identities is to "keep people away."[18] Keeping people away in a place like Ward's Island (in this case quite literally) can serve a number of functions for society: keep them away to protect worthier members of society from contagion; keep them away to protect "good people" in society from whatever dangers they are assumed to pose; keep them away so as not to be reminded of uncomfortable truths (e.g., that mental illness is part of life, that it can happen to anyone, and that our stressful competitive society has a number of social and psychological costs).[19] All of these functions remain largely unspoken in the modern discourse surrounding institutions such as psychiatric hospitals, homeless shelters, and community residences (except in places like internet message boards where people feel emboldened to anonymously say "the quiet part out loud"), but they are clearly present in the minds of policymakers, who dread community opposition and bad publicity.[20] This is by no means unique to New York City. The "not in my backyard" (NIMBY) phenomenon, in which local residents claim to recognize the importance of services such as clinics, congregate housing, or shelters but oppose their location in *their* neighborhood based on neutral concerns such as traffic and property values, was first described in the 1980s by Canadian researchers and continues to be a factor in policy decisions to this day.[21] A place like Ward's Island, which no longer (after the departure of my family and a few others in the early 1980s) has noninstitutional residents, presents an ideal way to steer clear of NIMBY issues, as there are no local residents to complain about the opening of a new shelter or residence.

Although institutional dumping is not unique to it, Ward's Island stands out among North American and European urban settings as a single geographic location in which so many institutions for marginalized persons are located next to each other. I have not been able to identify a comparable setting, located on an island, in any other major urban center in North America. Further, in many other cities, these institutions have been closed and services transitioned to other locations that are less distant from the urban center; for example, Philadelphia's Byberry State Hospital, located in a distant corner of the city and opened at roughly the same time as the New York City Asylum for the Insane, was closed in 1990.[22] At the same time, the simultaneous incorporation of the island as a place of recreation for New York City's more privileged residents within the past thirty years represents a contradiction that is also perhaps unique to New York: gentrification is pushing poorer residents further and further away from access to the city's resources that once offered some consolation from their poverty. In this way, New York City policymakers seem to want to "have it both ways" with a location such as Ward's Island, taking advantage of its remoteness for both recreation and institutional dumping.

The story of Ward's Island is an important but neglected part of the history of New York City. It is a history of New York's most marginalized citizens, predominantly immigrants and people of color, who were and are labeled as "insane" (or "mentally ill," in the modern version), shunned, and hidden away. Its story contains many of the themes of New York's history: immigration and xenophobia, rapid growth, public beautification, crime, drug crises, racism, overpolicing and "benign neglect," mass incarceration, abandonment of affordable housing and gentrification, the HIV and COVID-19 crises, and the struggle to develop systems to advance the public good. These themes, in turn, reflect larger issues that are relevant to many North American cities as well as cities in other parts of the world. It is also a case study of the U.S. mental health system, encompassing the start of the asylum movement, the rapid degradation of its lofty goals, the optimism of the early deinstitutionalization movement, the disappointments that quickly followed, the development of new evidence-based treatments and the recovery-oriented philosophy, and the struggle to find the best way to implement them, all within an overriding context of oppressive social systems, scarce resources, and public stigma. By telling the story of Ward's Island, I hope to create an account that is consistent with the aims of "restorative history," which seeks to "center communities that have experienced historical harm and exclusion."[23] I believe that the residents of Ward's Island have been just such a community.

In this book I discuss the history and development of Ward's Island and what it is now. My analysis is informed by several aspects of my personal identity: as a lifelong New Yorker who works in the public sector; as a descendent of immigrants from Greece; as a person of relative privilege (a white male from an upper-middle-class background) who is familiar with how more powerful segments of the city make decisions that protect their own interests; as a former Ward's Island resident and child of a longtime staff member; as an advocate and ally of the social movements of people with lived experience of mental health conditions; as a researcher who studies stigma toward people diagnosed with serious mental illnesses and has been involved in research on housing, community participation, and the development of evidence-based psychosocial treatments; and as a clinician who has been working with (and supervising trainees working with) formerly homeless persons diagnosed with serious mental illnesses for the past eighteen years. Using original data collection, I discuss the perspective of those who currently reside and work there as well as general New York City residents. I consider why Ward's Island has defied trends seen in other cities and persisted as a location of institutional dumping. Finally, I consider what Ward's Island can become—if New York City is willing to center the lives of the marginalized people who have long lived there.

2

WARD'S ISLAND

A Place Where No One Would Complain

Ward's Island's early recorded history is not dissimilar to that of other parts of New York City, with control passing from Native Americans to the Dutch and, eventually, to British colonizers.[1] Known as Tenkenas (which possibly means "uninhabited place") to Indigenous people, it was "purchased" in July 1637 by Wouter van Twiller of the New Netherland Company from Seyseys and Numers, chiefs of the Mayrechkeniackkingh tribe. Described as rich, arable, and fertile, it passed through the hands of a series of private owners of the merchant class throughout the Dutch and British colonial periods, including Thomas Delavall ("a receiver of shipping"), Thomas Parcell, the Bohanna family, and Benjamin Hildreth. During this time it was known alternately as Great Barrent or Great Barn Island. At some point in the late 1700s it was largely deforested, probably so that it could be used as an animal pasture.[2] As it sits along a strategic channel for entry into New York Harbor from Long Island Sound (originally called the "Helle-gat" by the Dutch, now called the Hellgate), it was fortified by the British during the American Revolution, from 1776 until the British Evacuation in 1783.[3] The meaning of the Dutch name Helle-gat, applied by the explorer Adriaen Block in 1614, is somewhat in dispute, because *hell* meant both "bright" and "fiery inferno" in Dutch; another theory is that this was a reference to the ancient Greek Hellespont (the Dardanelles Strait in modern-day Turkey). Most scholars seem to think that Block intended it to mean "gate of hell" because of the turbulence of the waters, as described in one early account: a "current sets so violently upon, that it threatens present shipwreck... and upon the Flood is a large Whirlpool, which continually sends forth a hideous roaring, enough to affright any stranger from passing further."

After the revolution, the island was incorporated into New York City and became known as Ward's Island, after its purchase by brothers Jasper and Bartholomew Ward in 1806. The Ward brothers were prominent merchants in New York City; Jasper Ward House, a building constructed in 1806, is still located at the corner of Peck Slip and South Street in the South Street Seaport historic district of Manhattan. The Ward brothers appeared to have had high hopes for the residential development of the island, establishing roads and separating the land into plots. They even arranged for the construction of a wooden bridge connecting the island to Harlem in 1807, as well as a ferry line, started in 1810, enabling prospective residents to commute to nearby Manhattan.[4] The bridge appears to have led to immediate complaints because it impeded navigation of the East River. Although it is unclear how long it remained in usable condition (one source states that it was destroyed in 1821), there is documentation that the bridge came to a definite end in December 1874, when it is reported to have been "carried away by the ice" floating in the East River. For whatever reason, residential development on the island did not take off as planned, and the island remained farmland, also serving as the site of a military fort (Fort Stephens) to defend New York Harbor during the War of 1812 and, after the war, a short-lived cotton factory (owned by the Belle Isle Factory Company).[5]

The end of the era of Ward's Island's private ownership and its beginning as the location of public institutions starts with an incident that it is chillingly reminiscent of modern NIMBYism. There was a dramatic rise in immigration from Ireland and Germany in the 1840s, linked to the Irish Potato Famine of 1845–1849 and the failed German democratic revolutions of 1848. As a result, in addition to the main immigrant receiving center at Castle Clinton in lower Manhattan, New York was charged with creating a place to house "sick and destitute emigrants, until they should be able to support themselves." In May 1847, the city found a suitable location for such an institution in an abandoned almshouse in the Long Island town of Astoria (presently a neighborhood in the borough of Queens), but an 1870s source states that the local "inhabitants, incensed at the project, assembled in disguise and destroyed the premises on the following evening."[6] Although no specific reason is given for why the local residents were so incensed as to destroy a public building, it seems likely that they were unhappy that thousands of "sick and destitute" foreign-born individuals would be living in their community. Shortly after this event, New York City immediately went to work on purchasing (at the price of $1,500/acre) 121 acres of Ward's Island facing the Manhattan waterfront (more than half of its total area). By December 1847 the land had been procured, and by 1848 the city had built a range of structures to house what would be known as the Emigrant Refuge and Hospital. The structures built included a refuge for the accommodation of up to 450 sick immigrants, a nursery for immigrant children (it is reported that between five and six hundred were housed there), a barracks to accommodate up to 1,200 immigrants (presumably those who were destitute but not sick), and a separate "lunatic asylum" for immigrants deemed insane, which is reported to have housed roughly 350 individuals in the 1860s. There are no reports of any widespread complaints or acts of vandalism toward the building of these institutions, intended to house more than 2,500 persons during a time when New York City's total population was roughly 313,000. It can be inferred that this was due to the remoteness of the island, which could only be reached by ferry.

Although its buildings had a stately appearance (see figure 2.1), there is evidence that the Emigrant Refuge and Hospital was managed in a strict manner, not unlike a correctional facility. An 1850 guide for the management of the institution described authority and responsibility residing with the "warden" of the facility and refers to the residents as "inmates."[7] Reports on the treatment of children indicate that harsh

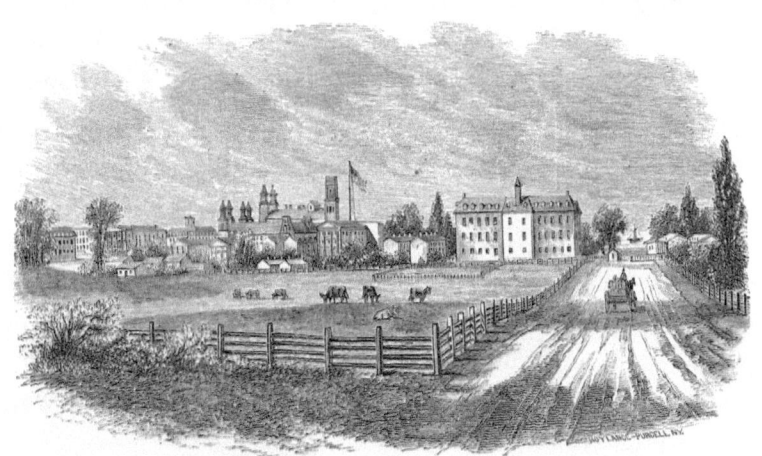

FIGURE 2.1 Emigrant Refuge and Hospital.

Source: New York Public Library Digital Collections.

discipline was used, noting that "the boys have a cowed way about them that is anything but pleasant."[8] The Emigrant Refuge and Hospital remained open until the 1890s, when the federal government took over the Emigration Department and Ellis Island was opened as a centralized location for managing the influx of immigrants.[9] However, as we shall see, Ward's Island continued to be a place where many immigrants would live.

Shortly after purchasing large parts of Ward's Island, New York City also found it a useful location for a different kind of "dumping"—the interment of the bodies of persons whose families could not afford to bury them (also known as a "potter's field"). New York began to bury large numbers starting in 1850 (exact estimates are unclear but it is likely that they numbered in the tens of thousands). A *New York Times* article in 1855 reported an "evil odor" emanating from roughly a quarter mile away from the location of the potter's field.[10] It was also reported that roughly one hundred thousand previously interred bodies were transferred to Ward's Island from the Manhattan potter's field in the area of what is now Washington Square Park in Greenwich Village.

City leadership envisioned other uses for the island and sought to purchase the rest of it in 1858. An 1858 article discussing Mayor Tiemann's efforts to do so clearly shows his concern that the city have the discretion to use the island as it saw fit: in response to a question regarding whether the city needed to own all of the island, the mayor replied "only that the City may have entire control over it."[11] The city, having learned from its experience trying to locate the Emigrant Refuge and Hospital in Astoria, was motivated to secure quick access to a location in which new institutions could be dumped.

By 1866, after an earlier act by the New York State Legislature, the city authorized the construction of a second institution—an Inebriate Asylum for persons who would now be considered to have alcohol dependence (see figure 2.2).[12] A structure that could accommodate four hundred "inebriates" was officially opened in late 1868.[13] Although it was initially designed to accommodate persons paying for the privilege of being kept away from alcohol, it gradually became focused on persons who could not contribute anything toward their treatment (presumably poor individuals, many of them likely immigrants).[14] Though the asylum initially followed a system of "exceedingly mild" rules, it eventually became much stricter, based on the perception that residents would abuse their freedom and continue to use alcohol even while residing at the asylum. Ultimately, it was believed that the Inebriate Asylum was unsuccessful in achieving its aims, and it was closed after only seven years in 1875.[15] After it closed, the building was briefly used to house a small Homeopathic Hospital that served indigent persons with a range of health conditions, including typhus and smallpox; it was described as "designed for the care of the city's poor." The Homeopathic Hospital moved to Blackwell's Island in 1894, when it was renamed Metropolitan Hospital, a name that lives on within New York City's public hospital system with a current location at First Avenue and Ninety-Seventh Street.

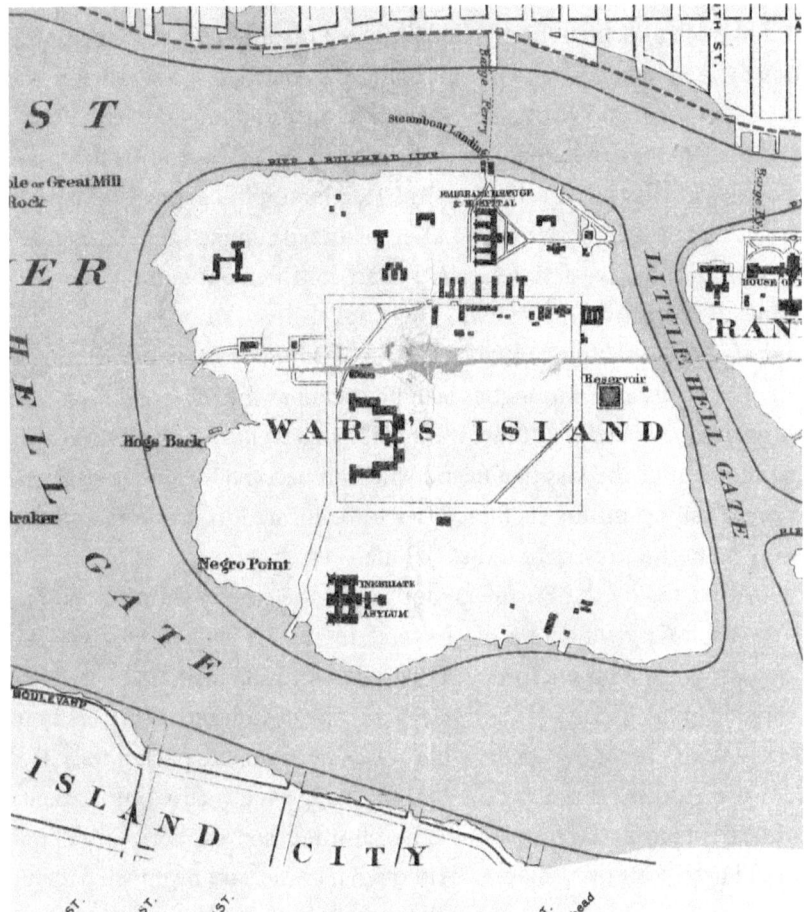

FIGURE 2.2 Ward's Island in the 1860s (Emigrant Refuge and Hospital located above and Inebriate Asylum located below).

Source: New York Public Library Digital Collections.

THE NEW YORK CITY ASYLUM FOR THE INSANE

The final institution to be opened on Ward's Island, and the one that would ultimately come to define it, was a branch of the New York City Asylum for the Insane (the predecessor to the present-day Manhattan Psychiatric Center), which opened in 1871. "Asylums" for people deemed to be insane (many of whom would be now diagnosed with mental disorders such as schizophrenia and bipolar I disorder, but also including those experiencing psychological conditions related to syphilis before the introduction of antibiotics) developed in France and England in the 1790s and early 1800s as a humane alternative to the warehousing of such individuals in jails and poorhouses. The treatment philosophy of the early asylums, called "moral treatment," emphasized compassion and engagement in productive activity, rather than confinement and harsh discipline.[16] "Moral treatment" was the English translation of *traitement moral*, developed in late 1700s (postrevolutionary) France by Philippe Pinel after his appointment as lead physician at the Bicetre Hospital in Paris. It is reported that Pinel was moved to develop a more humanistic approach after the loss of a friend who had become insane. It was considered important for such facilities to be located in pastoral settings, away from the stresses of industrial life.

Influenced by the European approach, the first asylum to open in New York City (and one of the first in the United States) was the Bloomingdale Asylum, in 1821, a private institution affiliated with New York Hospital, located at the present-day site of Columbia University in Manhattan's Morningside Heights area, then a remote part of the city.[17] However, as the Bloomingdale Asylum was privately run, only patients who could pay for their care could be admitted, so New York City's poor would need their own asylum.[18] Although it is unclear how much patients and families paid for care in the Bloomingdale Asylum, an 1888 critique asserting that it was not a public charity and should pay taxes estimated that the average cost was fourteen dollars per week per patient, or roughly two dollars per day (this is roughly six times the average daily cost of caring for patients in the public asylums in the late 1800s). New York City's first public asylum was opened on Blackwell's Island (now called Roosevelt Island), another East River island across from Manhattan, in 1839.[19] As previously discussed, it was recommended that asylums be located at least two miles away from urban areas, which was not practical within the constraints of Manhattan Island, so the location of the asylum on an island that could be accessed only by ferry provided an opportunity to "keep people away."[20]

As Stacy Horn has discussed extensively in *Damnation Island*, a history of the institutions on Blackwell's Island, although the New York asylums were theoretically based on the compassionate moral treatment philosophy of the early European asylums, the reality of how the city viewed their role can be seen in the fact that they were managed by the Department of Public Charities and Corrections and located on Blackwell's Island along with the city jail (precursor to the one currently on Riker's Island) and an almshouse for the homeless poor. This shared location indicated that the city viewed the East River island as a "one-stop shop" for the removal of society's undesirables. People charged with crimes were sometimes employed to serve as asylum attendants, given their availability on Blackwell's Island. As a result, although there were well-meaning individuals working within the asylum who intended to provide care and facilitate recovery, these intentions constantly struggled with the more dominant motive of "keeping people away" (discussed in chapter 1). As Horn has documented, conditions deteriorated very quickly on Blackwell's; only three years after its opening, Charles Dickens visited the facility while traveling in the United States and wrote that "everything had a lounging, listless, madhouse air" and that people lived in "naked ugliness and horror."[21] By the 1860s, the Blackwell's Island facility was becoming so overcrowded that it was decided it should house only women, and Ward's Island (just a small distance upriver) was selected as a site for male patients.

The best insight into what things were like at the Ward's Island branch of the New York City Asylum for the Insane comes from annual reports authored by its first long-term superintendent, Dr. Alexander MacDonald.[22] (The first two superintendents were Dr. M. G. Echeverria, who served from 1871 to 1872, and Dr. Theodore H. Kellogg, who served from 1872 to 1874, when Dr. MacDonald became superintendent.) Dr. MacDonald was fresh out of medical school and only twenty-six years old when he was appointed chief physician at the Ward's Island asylum in 1871.[23] By all accounts, he was an energetic and dedicated public servant, albeit one with a generally gloomy outlook on the potential for people labeled as insane to recover and return to the community (his reports include frequent mention of people being "incurable"). In his first report, written in 1874, he immediately began emphasizing several issues that would become recurring themes regarding the institution: it was overcrowded, poorly heated, understaffed (or staffed with underqualified individuals who might not treat the insane with appropriate compassion), and too inaccessible to allow for the regular delivery of necessary supplies (including mail from concerned family members) and/or regular engagement with the cultural resources of the city to provide "amusements" (such as music performances) for the patients. Buildings, though imposing and architecturally appealing in the Kirkbride (named after the Pennsylvania psychiatrist Thomas Story Kirkbride) style of many early asylums (see figure 2.3), were almost immediately considered to be in a poor state of repair, and care was observed to be underfunded.[24] MacDonald noted in his 1875 report that the average cost per patient was only thirty-three cents per day and, lest we wonder if this was a reasonable sum at the time, he explicitly stated "there is not a town or village upon this continent that spends as little upon its Insane as this great City of New York."[25] A 1916 report reflecting on the early history of the asylum corroborates MacDonald's assessment of poor conditions in even more forceful terms:

> The new Ward's Island building was faulty and inconvenient. Lighting and heating were inadequate. The attendants were too few, and food and clothing not much more than sufficient to keep soul and body together. The furniture was the rudest, benches without backs, deal tables that never saw a cloth, tin pannikins and iron spoons were the appointments, and the eating was frequently done with the fingers. Meal time meant bedlam. Many a patient went to bed with an ache in his stomach, and sedatives had to give the sleep which a full stomach would have found for itself. Nights were hideous with noises and profanity. Patients were locked in their rooms. The atmosphere was stifling. Straw-filled ticks, reeking and filthy, lay heaped about. Nurses were unknown and the attendants were coarse and inexperienced.[26]

There were, of course, advantages to locating the asylum on an island removed from the city, such as adequate space to keep patients engaged

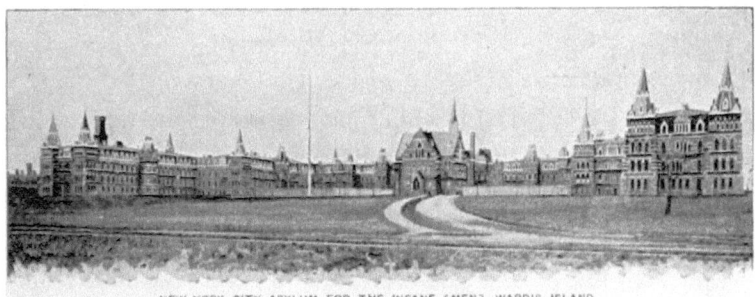

FIGURE 2.3 Ward's Island branch of New York City Asylum for the Insane in the late 1800s.

Source: Wikimedia Commons.

in worklike activity (a key to the moral treatment model) and the presence of water. The same source quoted above notes that Ward's Island boasted "a printing office, operated by compositors and pressmen from among the patients . . . brush, shoe and tailor shops . . . and every patient physically fit was put to work at his accustomed trade or in the farm and grounds." Running waters of the Hell Gate were also used to create a "a splendid sea bath with water from 5 to 2 ½ feet deep" from a cut "into the solid rock at the south end of the island" which allowed "as many as 1300 patients" to bathe at a time.[27]

Another major theme beginning in the earliest days of MacDonald's reports is that patients were predominantly immigrants, mostly from Germany and Ireland (half or more of the patients, depending on the year, were noted as "foreign born" throughout the late 1800s and early 1900s). The high proportion of foreign-born patients persisted even though "insane immigrants" were deported, as a matter of policy, if they were determined to be insane upon arrival in the United States. There was some controversy about how to carry out this policy. Initially, "insane aliens" were deported back to their country of origin on the first available ship without accompaniment. In 1907, new regulations required that they be accompanied by an attendant, but this turned out to be "too expensive" to carry out, so it was instead decided that the shipping company be "notified before sailing of the patient's condition."

The high number of immigrants at the asylum posed challenges in providing appropriate care to patients who did not speak English or were not Protestant. Ward's Island initially had only a Protestant chapel for patients to attend services, and MacDonald made a special request that Catholic services be initiated to accommodate the needs of (predominantly Catholic) Irish patients. In the early 1900s, the influx of patients from Eastern Europe (where my grandparents immigrated from at approximately this time) created new challenges with regard to religion, because many of these patients were Jewish or Eastern Orthodox. Later reports also spoke of linguistic issues as a barrier to the assessment of these immigrant patients.

The fact that immigrants were overrepresented among people housed at the asylum is consistent with a considerable body of evidence that immigration is a risk factor for what we now call schizophrenia (a major category of mental disorder that likely accounted for a large portion of what was called "insanity" in the late 1800s). A recent meta-analysis (a systematic quantitative review of studies) summarized this literature and found "substantial evidence for an increased relative risk of incidence [of schizophrenia] among first- and second-generation migrants compared to the native population," such that immigrants are roughly 1.7 times more likely to develop psychosis than native-born populations.[28] Based on the findings of the studies reviewed, the authors hypothesized that both "experienced discrimination and social exclusion," which act as sources of stress that affect brain chemistry, account for the consistent evidence for increased rates of schizophrenia among immigrants. Although these conclusions are based on research from the past twenty or so years, immigrants in the late 1800s and early 1900s undoubtedly experienced discrimination and social exclusion, and it is therefore plausible that similar processes may have affected rates of mental health conditions at that time. As has been extensively documented elsewhere, this period saw a rise in anti-immigrant sentiment throughout the United States.[29] This sentiment was fueled by the pseudoscientific justifications of the eugenics movement, which posited that Eastern and Southern Europeans (dismissed as "unemployed and unemployable human residuum" by one infamous and hugely popular work) were genetically inferior to "Nordic" Europeans.[30]

Absent from the official documentation regarding the asylum is any formal discussion of the race of patients, as charts only list "country of origin," and most Black New Yorkers would have been categorized as native-born at the time. (Records sometimes listed West Indies as a country of origin, with between zero and five patients listed with this as their country of origin.) One authoritative historical source suggests it is plausible that "blacks were discouraged from applying to mental hospitals" in New York in the late 1800s.[31] It is clear, however, that there were Black patients in the asylum, as race is mentioned in connection with some specific incidents; for example, a mention of the successful escape of a patient named Matthew Elliott noted that he was "colored," while a newspaper account from 1878 discussed the case of Henry H. Matthews ("colored man") and his wife's disagreement regarding whether he was insane. It is also known that Scott Joplin (the renowned Black American composer, originator of the ragtime style and many timeless pieces of music such as "The Entertainer") was hospitalized on Ward's Island in 1917 after developing syphilis and died there two months later.[32]

A dominant narrative among asylum superintendents in the post–Civil War period that would undoubtedly have affected Black patients on Ward's Island is the racist assumption that the "stresses" of freedom (related to the ending of the American system of slavery) had contributed to increased rates of "insanity" among Black Americans. As summarized by the historian Martin Summers in *Madness in the City of Magnificent Intentions*, there was a "proliferation of articles" in the 1870s and 1880s inferring a causal relationship between freedom and insanity among Black Americans, with paternalistic ideas about the childlike or animalistic nature of Black people featuring prominently in these influential accounts.[33] As late as 1916, a discussion of "inanity among the negroes" reflected these views, stating "it must be remembered that the negro is of a simple nature, giving little thought to the future . . . and desiring only the gratification of the present."[34] The treatment of Black patients would no doubt have been affected by these forms of "scientific" racism.

It is somewhat perplexing that the topic of how many Black patients were housed in the Ward's Island asylum, and *how* they were housed, is not mentioned in official reports, because we know that this issue had been discussed in psychiatry during the pre–Civil War years. In 1853, in an article titled "Asylums for Colored Persons," John M. Galt—the director of the country's first asylum in Virginia and cofounder of the Association of Medical Superintendents of American Institutions for the Insane (AMSAII), precursor to the modern-day American Psychiatric Association—wrote about whether and how "colored persons" should be housed in asylums and suggested that segregated units would be a viable option in states in which it was not feasible to build separate asylums (some southern states built entirely separate asylums for Black patients, such as Maryland's Crownsville).[35] Noting that New York and Pennsylvania had two of the largest communities of "colored persons," he specifically suggested that these states erect "a building for the purpose in the vicinity of an asylum, not within the same enclosure, but under the same directory and superintendence: or by appropriating an out-building or wing to this end; or simply by their admission into, the wards of white patients; care being taken in selecting the wards in which they are placed and distributed." We know that at least one other major urban asylum, Washington, DC's St. Elizabeth's, followed Galt's suggestion to create an entirely separate building for Black patients.[36]

While allowing that unsegregated units were possible, Galt also suggested that "mingling" Black patients with white patients could lead to problematic conflict between them. As a solution to this possibility, he proposed that they could be housed in wards with patients experiencing dementia, who might be less likely to react negatively to the Black patients.[37] We do not know if Ward's Island elected to follow Galt's suggestion of housing Black patients with white patients experiencing dementia, but it is certainly plausible. Based on a newspaper article from 1878, however, we can conclude with a fair degree of certainty that Ward's Island did *not* have segregated units. The article, which focuses on the killing of an attendant by a patient, describes how "William Scott, a colored patient" occupied the same room and slept "in adjacent beds" to "a German patient."[38] Despite clear evidence that Black patients were housed in the Ward's Island asylum, we can only speculate about what proportion of patients were Black and how the prevalent racism of the late 1800s and early 1900s may have affected their likelihood of being admitted, how they were diagnosed, and their treatment by staff and other patients in the facility.

Mistreatment of patients by staff is an issue that was regularly raised by MacDonald in his early reports, and his concern with it is suggested by a number of newspaper clippings regarding patient abuse in his personal archive. It makes sense that he would be especially sensitive to this issue because one of his predecessors, the briefly tenured (1871–1872) Dr. M. G. Echeverria, was removed from his position after there were "three cases of murder by brutal attendants."[39] MacDonald repeatedly discussed his struggles with being able to hire staff who were appropriately qualified to work with the insane, noting that the compensation was simply not adequate for the recruitment of qualified staff. Until 1875, attendants were primarily recruited from inmates at the city jail on Blackwell's Island, a practice that MacDonald seems to have brought to an end. However, this led to chronic understaffing and high turnover, with sixty staff leaving or being dismissed from their positions in 1875 alone.[40] The 1876 report noted a staffing ratio of one attendant per seventeen patients (this would be unacceptable by current standards, which define a safe patient-to-staff ratio as 1:4), and a salary of twenty dollars per month.

Despite MacDonald's efforts, newspaper accounts detail the brutal treatment of some patients by staff during his tenure, including an 1877 article in the *New York Herald* titled "A Brutal Keeper," which described how John Lowery, a "keeper" for the asylum, was charged with "brutally assaulting" an inmate named Rev. William Williams, and an 1878 article from an unidentified source discussing the criminal prosecution of an attendant Charles Mundinger for beating a patient.[41] One can only speculate as to how many more subtle incidents of mistreatment occurred that were not investigated or prosecuted.

A further concern noted in early reports is the issue of people being admitted to the asylum who were "not insane." In an early report MacDonald indicated that he had ordered the discharge of twenty-five patients categorized as "not insane"—some for feigning insanity to escape punishment, some intoxicated and only appearing insane, and some delirious due to a disease. In addition, he raised the possibility that relatives or others might seek to commit someone for inappropriate reasons, and in one case he noted "a possible suspicion of want of good faith in those committing him." In a later report, MacDonald decried efforts to essentially dump people who were not insane into the hospital—for example, to "transfer old and decrepit inmates of the almshouse who were not, within the meaning of the law, insane or proper subjects for hospital care." The issue of who was truly in need of detention at the asylum continued to be debated into the twentieth century, especially with regard to elderly persons experiencing what would now be labeled as poststroke dementia or Alzheimer's disease.

The patient population of the Ward's Island institution grew unabated between 1875 and the 1920s, reaching a highwater mark of 8,005 in 1930.[42] As can be seen in figure 2.4, the number of patients living there grew more than tenfold over a span of fifty years. Although this was partly the result of the institution's moving to accommodate both genders in the 1890s, as well as New York City's dramatic population growth over this period (from 1.2 million in 1880 to 6.9 million in 1930), the growth

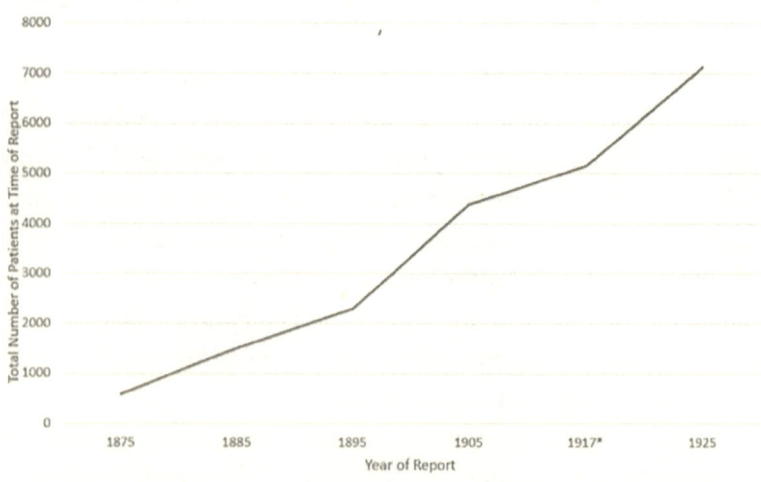

FIGURE 2.4 Annual census for Ward's Island Asylum/Hospital, 1875–1925.

in the patient population actually outpaced the city's population growth.[43] This was confirmed in general terms by calculations conducted in the 1930s by Benjamin Malzberg, who compiled statistical data across the state asylum system. Malzberg calculated the rate of patients per 100,000 for both New York City and New York State from 1909 to 1935 and found that this rate increased from 319 in 1909 to 505 in 1935 (an increase of more than 50 percent).[44] Although Malzberg could offer no explanation for this increase, it might perhaps have been due to the fact that the system was specifically designed to serve the poor and much of the city's population growth was from new immigrants who were arriving with minimal resources and therefore could be served only through public institutions if they experienced mental health conditions. (New York City's foreign-born population grew from roughly four hundred thousand in 1870 to more than two million in 1930.) Another factor may have been the rapid spread of syphilis, which often led to psychosis, and which was not successfully treated until penicillin became widely available in 1947. Although the steady expansion of the asylum (later hospital) was facilitated by the takeover of buildings previously used by the Inebriate Asylum (closed in 1875) and the Emigrant Refuge (closed in 1892), reports are clear that the asylum/hospital remained significantly overcrowded during this fifty-plus-year period, with reports in many years noting that it was roughly 40 percent over its stated maximum capacity. Reports also clearly indicated that overcrowding was detrimental to patients, with the 1920 report stating unequivocally that it was a "menace to the health of the patients."

SCANDAL AND ITS REPERCUSSIONS

Major changes occurred in the New York City Asylum in the 1890s that contributed to its growth and to some changes in its conditions. In 1886, the reporter Elizabeth Jane Cochrane (pen name Nelly Bly) published an account based on her experience in the Blackwell's Island asylum, where she feigned insanity to gain admission (later compiled in her book

Ten Days in a Madhouse).⁴⁵ Her report detailed horrific living conditions and treatment, prompting public outcry and scrutiny over the conditions within the asylum. Though the exposé did not specifically address Ward's Island, it was a bombshell that created ripples felt farther up the East River. We know that the management of the Ward's Island asylum was sensitive to this, as MacDonald mentioned it in his 1887 report. Five years later, in 1892, there was an internal investigation of conditions in both asylums and a report published by the City Advisory Commission on Care of the Insane. This report determined that conditions were "pitiable" on Blackwell's Island but considerably better on Ward's Island and recommended that all of the city's "insane" (including women) be transferred to Ward's Island.⁴⁶ The report also recommended increased funding for their care and the removal of substandard accommodations such as a straw mattresses, as well as separation of the care of the insane from other public charities. The report's recommendations were accepted, and there was a gradual transfer of female patients to Ward's Island, facilitated by the use of recently vacated buildings from the State Emigrant Refuge.

A period of change on Ward's Island was only just starting, however. Only two years later, on May 13, 1894, the *New York Herald* published an exposé of conditions in the Ward's Island asylum that would lead to further shakeups. The article, based on an insider report from a young female physician, made a range of allegations, including insufficient clothing and food, incompetent attendants, prevalent disease, and poor bathing facilities. MacDonald rebuked it as a "work of fiction" in his own 1894 report, but his statement rings hollow given that he had been regularly complaining of these same issues in his annual reports throughout the previous two decades. The *New York Herald* article led to further investigations, this time by a state commission. Although the commission determined that there was no negligence and absolved MacDonald of blame, it concluded that New York City should no longer be responsible for management of the public care of the insane and that control of the asylum should pass to New York State, as state institutions "represent all that is best in the present state of knowledge respecting the care and treatment of the insane."

Despite some resistance from New York City's government, due in large part to fiscal considerations too intricate to detail here, the writing was on the wall. Control of the Ward's Island asylum was transferred to New York State in 1896, with its name officially changed to Manhattan State Hospital. This name change was considered to reflect the more humane and modern sensibilities with which the state was aligned. Dr. MacDonald remained the superintendent until 1904, when he retired "after thirty years of service" and the direction of the hospital passed to Dr. William Mabon, and later Dr. Marcus Heyman.

Change in management and name notwithstanding, there is not much evidence for any substantial change in the conditions at the newly dubbed Manhattan State Hospital following the state takeover.[47] Annual reports written by hospital superintendents still noted that the hospital was overcrowded and remote (still only accessible by aging ferries), that buildings were in a poor state of repair, that it was underfunded, and that it was difficult to hire qualified staff due to inadequate compensation (the 1919 report explicitly stated: "raise the wage and you will raise the number of workers"). Difficulties in commuting to work on the island led to the building of housing for some staff during these years, including the house that my family would end up moving into in 1970.

Becoming a state institution allowed Manhattan State Hospital to sometimes send patients away to other (often distant) state institutions to reduce overcrowding, which it could not do as a city asylum. Although it is not clear why specific patients would be transferred, it is plausible that they may have been selected if they lacked family connections within New York City. In a study of the lives of people at the Willard State Hospital in New York State's Finger Lakes region, authors Darby Penney and Peter Stastny discuss how a group of 116 patients were transferred (by train) from Manhattan State Hospital to Willard in 1919.[48] One of these patients, profiled in detail in the book, was an immigrant from Germany named Theresa Lehner who had previously served as a nun before leaving a convent for unknown reasons. Lehner lacked family connections within New York City, perhaps making her a preferred candidate for transfer to a hospital roughly 250 miles away from her adopted home.

A tragic event in February 1923 that brought home the poor condition of Manhattan State Hospital's buildings was the outbreak of a fire in an old building in a hospital ward that was greatly overcrowded, killing twenty-five people (twenty-two patients and three attendants). The annual report in which it was discussed described it as "the greatest tragedy in the history of the State institutions for the care of the insane." In addition to the age and condition of the building, a contributing factor was the fact that firefighters had to travel to the island from Manhattan via boat with hastily gathered equipment.[49] In response to the event, Governor Al Smith stated: "the fact is unquestionably known ahead of time that many buildings used for the housing of the wards of the state are old, out-of-date and impossible of improvement to the point where safety from fire can in any degree be guaranteed." As a result, the state legislature approved a fifty-million-dollar bond issue to improve the physical plant of the "out-of-date" buildings, which gradually led to improvement in the hospital's structures.

There is no evidence for any reduction in overcrowding, however, as it continued to be decried in reports from 1924 through 1930. The 1928 report specifically discussed the detrimental effects of overcrowding on patients from a perspective that suggests the development of a more modern sensibility, consistent with what would predominate when deinstitutionalization began roughly thirty years later: "It is far more costly to maintain an unrecovered patient in a State hospital for the remainder of life than it is to increase capital investment . . . not only are humanitarian interests unserved, but actual extravagance results when patients theoretically recoverable are not restored to society." Relatedly, one new development starting in 1906 and increasing thereafter was the practice of offering patients "parole," enabling them to live in the general New York community (most likely with family members) while remaining under the supervision of the hospital for a period of six months, at which point they would be officially discharged. The practice continued to operate to a limited extent (with only a few hundred out of a several thousand patients being offered this opportunity) throughout the prewar years.

Another change that can be seen starting to slowly develop was an increasingly medical view of the patients. Shortly after the state takeover,

Dr. Adolf Meyer, an immigrant from Switzerland who would come to have a tremendous impact on American psychiatry, was appointed the director of the New York State Pathological Institute (a research institute associated with the state hospital system), and he elected to open a research laboratory in an abandoned bakery on Ward's Island.[50] During his brief tenure (between 1901 and 1908), the institute served as a training site for the physicians who worked in New York's state hospitals, establishing practices such as the writing of progress notes and the use of new diagnostic categorization systems that had been developed in Europe. Meyer's influence can be seen in the fact that, in 1905, the terms *psychosis* and *dementia praecox* (the diagnostic category created by the German psychiatrist Emil Kraepelin at the turn of the century that would eventually be known as schizophrenia) were used for the first time. From then on, reports began discussing the proportion of patients admitted who met criteria for various diagnostic categories, including dementia praecox and manic-depression (now called bipolar disorder). Further, increasing reference is made to various forms of treatment, including occupational therapy (engagement in work-related activities, consistent with the principles of moral treatment) and hydrotherapy (which involved full body immersion in warm baths to help calm patients). Although the development of psychopharmacological agents was decades away, at least in spirit the state hospital was beginning to view itself as a place of treatment for mental illness rather than of indefinite confinement for the incurably "insane." This likely also reflected Meyer's influence, as he was intent on establishing psychiatry's legitimacy as a medical discipline and would eventually coin the term *psychobiology* to describe his theories of how physiological forces affected the mind.

Despite these changes, there is not much evidence that things were significantly different on Ward's Island in the 1920s than in the 1870s. The hospital had the island largely to itself, and although it kept expanding, it remained overcrowded as the patient census continued to outpace its expansion. Life on Ward's Island was about to change in the 1930s, however, as it was about to come into contact with one of the most influential and forceful personalities of the twentieth century: "master builder" Robert Moses.

3

PARKLAND OR INSTITUTIONAL DUMPING GROUND?

After it was acquired by New York City in 1847, Ward's Island remained remote and reachable only by ferry. This was advantageous from the city government's perspective because it minimized community opposition to the constant growth of the institutions located there, but it created challenges for the transport of staff to the institutions and the provision of services and goods to their residents. In the era between the First and Second World Wars, however, it became apparent that Ward's Island would soon be physically connected to New York City and might no longer be used to house institutions, as it had for the previous eighty years.

The first step toward connection between Ward's Island and the larger world came in the 1910s, with the construction of the New York Connecting Railroad Bridge, better known as the Hell Gate Bridge. Authorized by statute in 1900, commissioned in 1912, and constructed in 1916, the bridge provided a route for trains from the New York, New Haven and Hartford Railroad Company to travel from New England to New York's Pennsylvania Station (on Manhattan's West Side). The bridge allowed trains to avoid going through Manhattan Island by going over Randall's and Ward's Islands into Astoria, Queens, before proceeding into Manhattan through a tunnel under the East River.

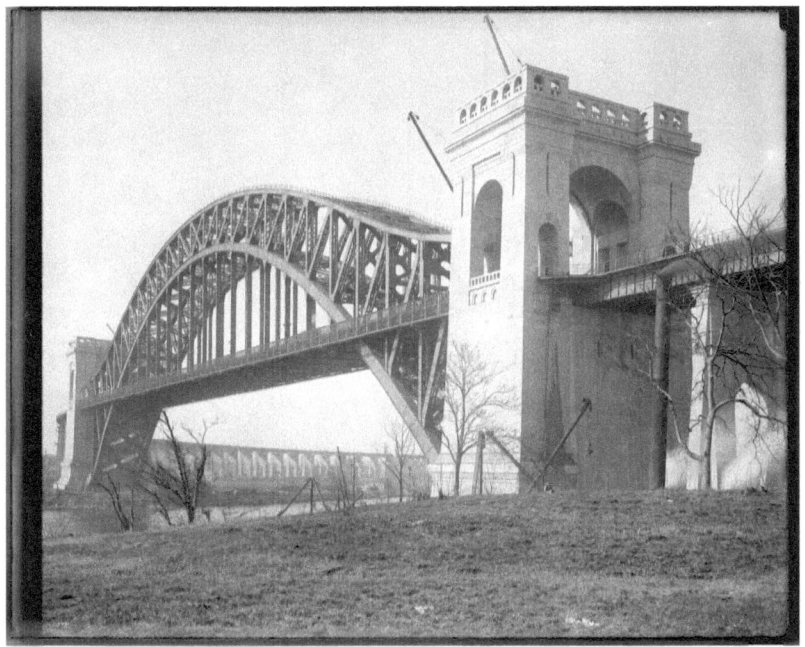

FIGURE 3.1 The completed Hell Gate Bridge in 1917.

Source: U.S. Library of Congress.

The bridge was, and is, an architectural marvel, visible from both Manhattan and Queens, and one that many find appealing to this day (see figure 3.1).

Despite the sense of psychological connection that the Hell Gate Bridge undoubtedly provided, it still offered no access to Ward's Island, as there was no train station on the island and no pedestrian paths were built that might allow people to traverse it by foot.[1] One can imagine that it gave island residents a "so close but so far" feeling as they remained unable to reach the mainland except by boat. As a child growing up on the island—even though there was road access by that time—I can certainly recall being amazed and fascinated by the impressive Hell Gate Bridge in a way that is consistent with this perspective.

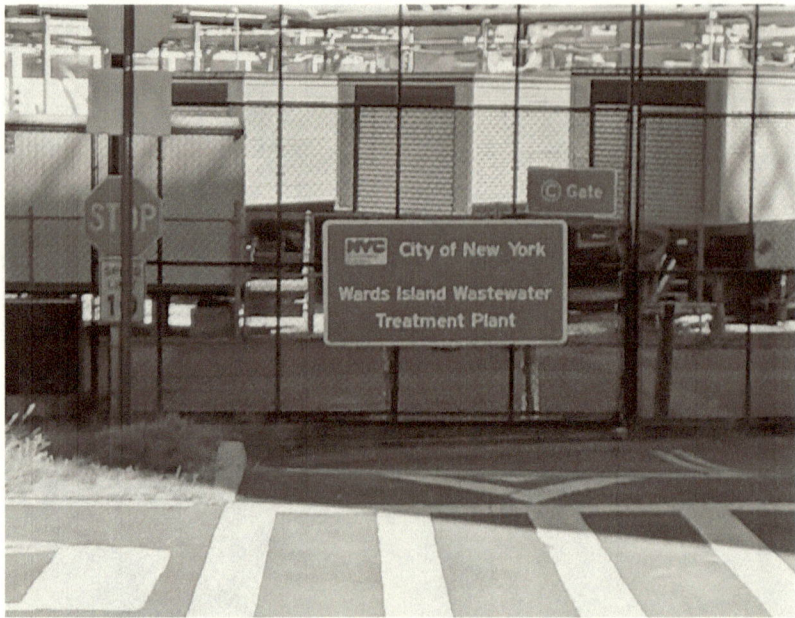

FIGURE 3.2 Entrance to the Ward's Island Wastewater Treatment Plant, September 26, 2022.

Source: Photo by author.

In 1927 a portion of the eastern side of the island was acquired by New York City, by special authorization of the New York State Legislature, to house a new type of "dumping" facility considered too noxious to house elsewhere: a wastewater treatment plant. Completed in 1937, this facility, the first of its kind in New York City (and one of only three "major" sewage treatment facilities in the world in 1939), processes a substantial portion of New York City's sewage to this day (see figure 3.2).[2] Although the land for the wastewater treatment facility was acquired by the city with the approval of the state legislature, it is clear from the 1927 and 1928 Manhattan State Hospital annual reports that the directors of the hospital were upset about ceding part of the island's area for this type of project and made no bones about their opposition.[3]

CONVERSION TO CITY PARK?

Even as the wastewater treatment facility was being built, more dramatic changes were in the air regarding the future of Ward's Island. In 1926 an association of policymakers and business leaders, operating under the auspices of the Regional Plan Association of New York, issued a recommendation that Ward's and Randall's Islands be converted into public parks and their existing institutions be removed.[4] The question of where hospital patients would go did not seem to greatly concern the planners, who assumed that they could be moved to locations beyond the city limits. The allure of Ward's Island as parkland is clearly evident from figure 3.3 (which was developed by planners), showing that the substantial acreage of Ward's Island, if accessible, could provide significant recreational opportunities for Manhattan residents.

This recommendation had a number of powerful allies, including newly elected New York governor (and future U.S. president) Franklin D. Roosevelt, who stated in 1929: "it is essential that provision be made for moving the state institutions off Ward's Island and Randall's Island so that these islands may be returned to the city for recreational use and other city purposes." He further linked this recommendation to the idea that the hospital had outgrown its island setting and needed to be moved to a larger location: "the 1927 provision [to create the Wastewater Treatment Facility] was made by special act for releasing part of the hospital grounds at Ward's Island to the city for the construction of a sewage disposal plant. This limited the area for outdoor recreation for the inmates of the hospital.... The hospital is overcrowded and is gradually being forced off the island."[5]

Although Governor Roosevelt's statement of intent to evict Manhattan State Hospital was clearly important, in the late 1920s a figure emerged with even more direct influence on the physical landscape of the New York City region: Robert Moses. Though never elected to office, Moses nevertheless wielded tremendous power and influence in New York State and City, roughly from 1924 to 1964, holding multiple appointed titles simultaneously in addition to chairing "authorities"

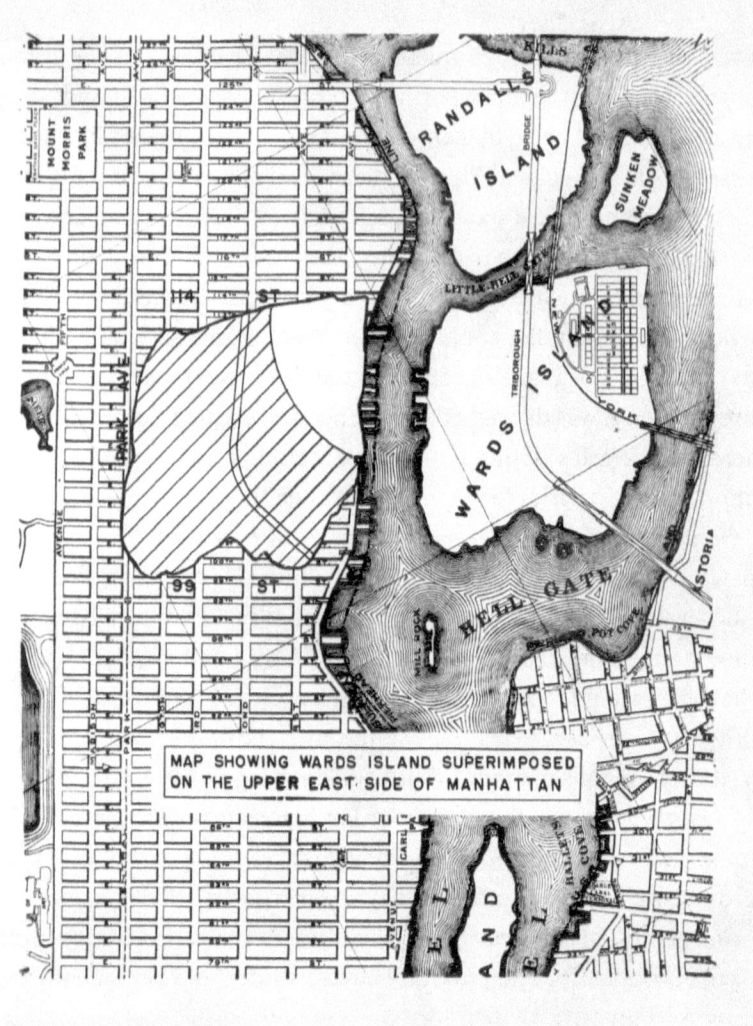

FIGURE 3.3 Map of Ward's Island, 1937, emphasizing its size and potential to provide recreational space.

Source: New York Public Library Digital Collections.

(quasi-corporate public entities with direct control of millions of dollars in funds raised through fares and tolls).[6] His penchant for evicting people from their residences in order to build roadways has been well documented. In the 1920s Moses was already both Long Island Parks Commissioner and chair of the New York State Council of Parks and was revered for having created Jones Beach State Park on Long Island's south shore. Moses added his voice to the chorus supporting the idea that Ward's Island should be turned into parkland. By the early 1930s he had linked this idea to his interest in road building with the ambitious proposal to build a series of bridges connecting Manhattan, Queens, and the Bronx, with Ward's and Randall's Island's as platforms, which would become known as the Triborough Bridge project.[7]

Rapid movement toward these dual goals was facilitated by two factors: (1) the availability of federal New Deal funds (courtesy of then President Franklin Roosevelt's administration) for the completion of large-scale public works projects, as a way of addressing widespread unemployment during the Great Depression; and (2) the election of Fiorello LaGuardia as New York City mayor in 1933. LaGuardia, whose candidacy Moses had allied himself with, wanted to include the popular Moses in his administration. However, Moses made it clear that his participation would be contingent on being granted "unified control of the whole metropolitan system of parks and parkway development." LaGuardia complied and appointed him both the city's inaugural parks commissioner and the chief executive officer of the Triborough Bridge Authority. Moses continued to hold his statewide positions even as he moved into these city positions, and his influence at the state level appears also to have served him in his goal to turn Ward's Island into parkland. New York State mental hygiene officials were opposed to the closure of Manhattan State Hospital, but Moses "persuaded [Governor] Lehman to overrule the state officials." Although the Triborough Bridge Authority funds were not intended to support parks, Moses convinced federal authorities to allow him to use those funds for the creation of the park facilities on Ward's and Randall's Islands.[8]

Movement toward construction of the bridge and the transfer of institutional residents proceeded rapidly and firmly thereafter. In its 1931 report, Manhattan State Hospital's director voiced an awareness of a "growing idea that the hospital is to be evacuated within a few years, and that the Island will be reclaimed by the city of New York," and within two years the hospital was aggressively transferring patients to other state hospitals. Its census declined for first time in its history, with the transfer of nearly two thousand patients to "other institutions for the insane" in anticipation of their soon being driven from the island.

By 1933 it became official state law that the hospital "be evacuated" within ten years and that "inmates [be] transferred to other state hospitals and the lease of the land by the City of New York to the State of New York be terminated after such transfer." Specifically, "the department of mental hygiene is hereby directed within ten years after the taking effect of this act, to remove the inmates of Manhattan state hospital, now located on Ward's Island, and such property and equipment used in or in connection with such hospital, as it may desire, to the Pilgrim state hospital on Long Island, or to other state hospitals, in which it shall establish suitable quarters and accommodations for them." It was also made clear that there should be no trace left of the old institutional buildings of Ward's Island: "The city of New York shall proceed as soon as possible after the governor shall have so certified to the mayor, as provided in section four of this act, to raze all of the buildings, structures and other improvements of the Manhattan state hospital."[9]

The proposed relocation of patients from Ward's Island could be considered a new form of dumping, facilitated by the automobile age and the sense that distances of fifty or more miles were no longer a concern (before the realization that traffic could clog roads, making travel much less straightforward than expected). There appears to have been little consideration of how the relocation of hospital patients—by definition New York City residents—to suburban state hospitals in Suffolk County (on Long Island), Rockland County, or Dutchess County (both north of the city) would affect the patients' ability to remain in contact with friends and family members or to be supported while in the community "on parole." Moses and his allies at the time pitched the choice as being between decrepit institutional buildings for patients and parks for the people of Manhattan and the Bronx. As Moses put it in a memorandum from the 1930s, turning Ward's Island into a park would address the "deplorable shortage of space for active play on the upper part of Manhattan Island and the lower part of the Bronx . . . development of play facilities will solve this problem, and . . . it can be solved in no other way."[10] The assumption seems to have been that state hospital patients would be lifetime residents, and proximity to family, friends, and communities of origin was therefore not important. The emerging philosophy (seen in the writings of hospital superintendents discussed in the previous chapter) that reentry into the community was possible, desirable, and potentially facilitated by a supervised transitional period seems not to have reached the consciousness of state-level policymakers at the time.

With legal hurdles cleared, Moses went to work rapidly on construction of the Triborough Bridge overpass, which opened in 1935. Institutions on Randall's Island that lay in the preferred path of the overpass, including a children's hospital (which was operated by New York City and therefore did not require negotiation with the state), were immediately evicted. Meanwhile, the car-oriented Moses seems to have been interested in ensuring that the newly constructed automobile bridge would be the only way of getting on and off the island. He first created a "a low-level bridge between Randall's and Ward's Island so that vehicles bound for Ward's Island can use the Randall's Island ramp," noting that "this bridge is of course of great advantage to the state institutions on Ward's Island." Afterward, in a letter dated November 14, 1934, he requested that the 116th Street ferry to Ward's Island be discontinued immediately after completion of the bridge and that arrangements be made for "a necessary road and parking system on Ward's Island." Ward's Island would no longer be disconnected from Manhattan Island, but now it would be accessible only by vehicle. In place of the long-standing ferry transporting patients directly from Bellevue Hospital, two ambulances were now dedicated to patient transportation. Soon after, a public bus was established, which, according to a 1937 hospital report,

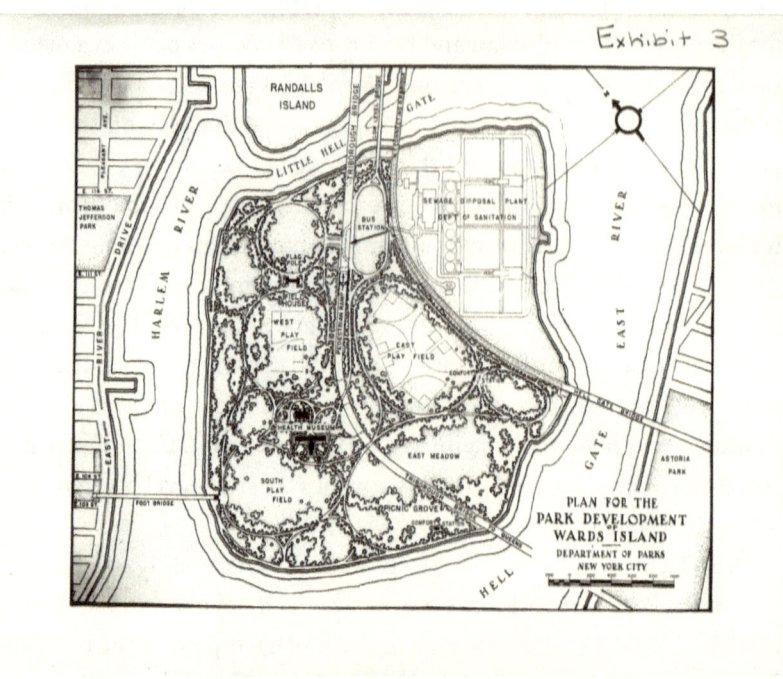

FIGURE 3.4 Rendering of plans for Ward's Island Park, 1937.

Source: New York City Municipal Archives.

"affords opportunity through a five-cent fare for visitors and employees to leave Lexington Avenue and 125th Street and reach the hospital via Randall's Island at maximum intervals of one-half hour. . . . It has been reasonably satisfactory."[11]

Plans for parkland development were ambitious but proceeded much more slowly than the construction of roadways (see figure 3.4). The original 1937 plans promised that a pedestrian bridge would be built so that East Harlem residents could access the island's parks on foot (they also included provision for a "health museum," which I have not seen discussed elsewhere). However, ground was not broken for the bridge until 1949, and construction was not completed until 1951. It is unclear how many New York residents elected to take the bus to Ward's Island for recreation or exploration during the 1930s and 1940s.

CHANGE AT MANHATTAN STATE HOSPITAL

Annual reports from the hospital in the 1930s indicate a rapid reduction in the hospital census immediately preceding and following the passage of the Laws of 1933, Chapter 144.[12] The 1933 report noted that the hospital census had been cut in half in the span of four years, declining from more than eight thousand in 1930 to fewer than four thousand in 1933. Where were the patients going? This was not what would later be known as deinstitutionalization, with patients transitioning to community-based settings, but rather "trans-institutionalization," with the overwhelming number of patients being transferred to Pilgrim State Hospital, in Suffolk County, approximately fifty miles from Manhattan; other, similarly distant, transfer destinations included Harlem Valley State Hospital in Dutchess County, Rockland State Hospital in Rockland County, and Kings Park State Hospital, also in Suffolk County.[13]

Annual reports made it clear that these mass transfers were being conducted under duress and were not viewed as beneficial to patients. For example, the 1935 report asserted that "there should be a State hospital easily accessible from the boroughs of Manhattan and Bronx to accommodate those patients who for financial or other reasons cannot be readily visited by their families," noting that "as it is the policy of the State not to unduly isolate the insane, it would seem to be consistent with that policy to afford care and treatment for the group mentally disordered, whose immediate relatives are actually unable to visit them at comparatively distant points." The 1936 report further stated: "it is obvious that it is a great source of satisfaction to the relatives and friends of patients to be able to reach [their loved ones] at small cost and time . . . a large number of these friends express themselves unable, particularly financially, to visit patients at a distance from these boroughs." The benefit of the accessibility of the hospital for the potential discharge of patients to the community ("parole") was also noted: "a factor in maintaining [a 15 percent] parole rate is the nearness of the hospital to the metropolitan area which facilitates the visits of relatives who in many cases who would find it a hardship to visit a more distant hospital. Many of them are eager to take home their sick ones soon after admission." These points about the benefits of having a hospital located close to patient's community of origin would be reiterated again and again throughout the 1930s and 1940s.

Despite dramatic reductions, the decline eventually slowed and the patient population actually began to increase slightly. In 1936, the population fell below three thousand, then rose to roughly 3,500 and remaining between three and four thousand until the early 1950s. Robert Moses complained to the press in 1934 that the hospital seemed to be dragging its feet: "Why they've had four years now $250,000 available for the purchase of a site and they haven't done a thing."[14] World War II would soon become a factor, but even before the war the stalling of the rapid rate of transfer seems to have been more related to the large-scale influx of a new type of patient: elderly persons with various forms of dementia. The 1937 report noted that the majority of the patients being admitted were "old and infirm, and unsuitable to be sent to a distant hospital," implying that they would be at risk if transported to Pilgrim, Rockland, or Harlem Valley State. Admissions data indicate that roughly 60–70 percent of people admitted during these years were over sixty. Aside from the mainstay dementia praecox (schizophrenia), two of the three largest diagnostic categories for new admissions during this period were "psychosis with cerebral arteriosclerosis" and "senile psychosis."[15] These two conditions, related to stroke and dementias such as Alzheimer's, would not now be seen as appropriate justifications for admission to a state psychiatric hospital; they would be viewed as appropriate for home care, assisted living with support, or nursing care. In the 1930s, however, these types of facilities were not widely available, so the state psychiatric hospital seems to have become the go-to placement for the indigent elderly of New York City.

Hospital administrators voiced the view that the influx of elderly patients represented the "dumping" of a group that was not appropriate for admission to a state hospital. After becoming director in 1942, the superintendent Dr. John Travis did not hesitate to editorialize on this topic in his reports, stating that "able-bodied patients are becoming fewer and fewer as the years roll by and some of the wards are beginning to take on the coloring of an Old Folks Home"; in a later report, he stated that "the conclusion is inescapable that some families of these elderly patients are unwilling to have them in their homes, even when they can provide space for them." Despite Dr. Travis's judgmental tone, it is certainly plausible that the shift was related to the financial struggles that the low-income families served by the hospital were enduring during the Great Depression, which made it more challenging for them to support elderly relatives.

The influx of elderly patients does not appear to have altered other demographic characteristics of the patient population. Consistent with data reported since the late 1800s, annual reports throughout the 1930s and 1940s noted that approximately 50 percent of patients were foreign born. Unfortunately, there was still no information provided on the racial characteristics of patients during this period. However, there is evidence from annual reports that Black patients continued to be treated at Manhattan State Hospital. In the 1937 report there was a discussion of a research project at the hospital on "blood groups in 'constitutional psychoses'" that included the construct of race for the first time, mentioning a "mixed race," a "colored race," and a "Hebrew race." In addition to reflecting the eugenic ideas popular at the time, this indicates that, despite not reporting on it in official data, the hospital management thought of the patients as belonging to racial groups characterized by skin tone as well as religion. As I have elsewhere discussed, the eugenics movement, which viewed mental illness as an indication of "defective" traits that should be eradicated from the national gene pool, exerted a powerful influence on American psychiatry in the early twentieth century, leading to the enactment of forced sterilization laws in forty states and influencing Nazi Germany's more radical "euthanasia" policy.[16]

Further confirmation that "Negroes" represented a significant proportion of the state hospital population in New York State comes from a study by Benjamin Malzberg that used combined data from all state hospitals in the late 1930s. This study found more than 3,900 admissions of Black patients to state psychiatric hospitals between July 1, 1938 and June 30, 1941 and, after comparing rates of admission to those of white patients, concluded: "it appears clear that Negroes had higher rates of first admissions than whites to hospitals for mental disease in New York State."[17] While the scientific soundness of this conclusion is questionable by contemporary standards (especially given the socioeconomic bias of those who were served by the state hospital system), it nevertheless demonstrates that Black patients constituted a significant portion of the patient population at Manhattan State Hospital. Also of note, dementia praecox (the diagnosis that would eventually be renamed schizophrenia) was the leading diagnostic reason for admission among Black patients (accounting for 45 percent of admissions), a rate that exceeded that of white patients (27 percent), which Malzberg believed could be explained on the basis of "migration and environment."[18] Though based on conjecture, Malzberg's broad-based hypothesis is consistent with recent research findings, which indicate that risk for psychosis is elevated among Black individuals who live in societies where they have been historically marginalized (including the United Kingdom and North America) and that "structural racism" affects the risk for schizophrenia and related psychoses through a range of environmental mechanisms, including "neighborhood factors, cumulative trauma and stress, and prenatal and perinatal complications."[19]

Parallel to the story of Manhattan State Hospital's struggle to stay open, reports during the 1930s and 1940s document a fundamental change in the types of "treatment" being offered to patients. In reports prior to 1937, the predominant modes of treatment were hydrotherapy and occupational therapy. Occupational therapy, descended from the moral treatment of the early asylums, was described as follows: "through the medium of prescribed work and recreation, a constant effort is made to rehabilitate sick minds and direct them towards a more normal and social behavior"; it was characterized as the main therapeutic activity of the hospital. However, starting in 1937, occupational therapy and hydrotherapy were decreasingly discussed and new somatic methods began to be introduced—specifically, insulin shock therapy (which induces a seizure, paradoxically leading to a reduction in symptoms), as well as the prescription of medications such as Metrazol (a stimulant) and barbiturates. (Antipsychotic medications did not become available until the 1950s.) Electric shock therapy, a precursor to modern-day electroconvulsive therapy (ECT), was introduced in 1942, as were other medications.

By 1943 there was almost no discussion of occupational therapy in the hospital's annual reports, and in 1950 hydrotherapy was said to be no longer practiced because of a lack of trained personnel and a water shortage. At roughly the same time, a unit dedicated to conducting what would now be seen as the barbaric practice of psychosurgery was established for the first time in 1949. Although lobotomy, involving the severing of connections in the brain's prefrontal cortex by way of skull puncture, is the best-known form of psychosurgery, hospital records indicate that topectomy (which involves the removal of portions of the frontal cortex) was also practiced.

The move away from the more traditional activity-based treatments toward more somatic and surgical approaches may be linked to a number of factors. The graying of the patient population meant that patients were less able to be engaged in worklike activities, the focus of occupational therapy. At the same time, the United States' entry into World War II meant that, as staff left to join the war effort, the hospital became even more understaffed than previously. This made staff-intensive approaches like occupational therapy difficult to maintain. Parallel to this was the increase in the medical identity of physicians who managed the hospital. The field of psychiatry, as it is now known, did not officially exist until the 1920s. What is now the American Psychiatric Association was originally called the Association of Medical Superintendents of the American Institutions for the Insane, suggesting that it was primarily a management-oriented position.[20] In the 1910s, Adolf Meyer (who, as we saw in chapter 2, briefly worked on the grounds of Manhattan State Hospital after the turn of the century), helped create the field of psychiatry with a decidedly biological bent while at the Phipps Psychiatric Clinic at Johns Hopkins University (in Baltimore, Maryland). With increasing medical identity and a desire to be legitimized as a medical profession came the search for more somatic methods to address mental illness.

While somatic approaches were increasingly being used, there was some mention of more contemporary psychosocial treatments, though they appear to have occupied a fairly marginal corner of what the hospital provided. The first Alcoholics Anonymous meeting among patients is reported to have occurred on December 18, 1947, with the statement that "insofar as these meetings have progressed it can be reported that a limited number of patients have benefited."[21] In the same year, it was reported that a psychology department had been started, staffed by a single psychologist (John Smith), with the initial use of projective psychological testing approaches including the Roschach and the Thematic Apperception Test (names that would still be familiar to present-day psychologists).

A FINAL REPRIEVE

As the reduction of the patient census at Manhattan State Hospital stalled with the influx of elderly patients, the state passed a bond issue in 1937 providing for funding to build a new state hospital. In its annual report, the hospital directors made a plea for a new hospital to be built at an already available location: Ward's Island. They noted that "the board has already registered its belief that the institution should continue on Ward's Island and now earnestly reiterates a recommendation that this be carried out by law. It is the conclusion of the board that the interests of the mentally-ill patients are such that they should not be superseded by the interests of the city in extending its park system to include Ward's Island." It is likely that state government officials were beginning to hear these pleas, and the beginning of World War II provided a justification for listening to them. Although the Laws of 1933 had required that the hospital be completely vacated by 1943, the Laws of 1941, Chapter 717, provided a five-year extension, permitting the hospital to function until April 7, 1948. At the same time, a sum of $300,000 was granted for the "remodeling and reconditioning" of the hospital building, an unusual investment for buildings scheduled to be demolished within seven years. In 1941 a state hearing was held in which a range of psychiatric experts testified about the impacts that closing the hospital would have on the New York community.[22] In 1944, as the end of the war drew near, the hospital superintendent suggested there would soon be an increased need for the treatment of mental illness (presumably due to combat trauma), warning that "in view of the looming postwar problems from a psychiatric point of view, every available bed will be required to minister to presently foreseeable situations."[23]

Meanwhile, conditions at Manhattan State Hospital were judged to be dire. In an unannounced visit to the hospital conducted in the early 1940s, reported originally in the *New York Post* and later included in his 1948 book *The Shame of the States* (in a chapter titled "New York's Isle of Despair"), the journalist Albert Deutsch noted that "the present institution is in an appalling state of deterioration and disrepair as a result of years of neglect in expectation of abandonment." He added that several wards were "in indescribable stages of filth and general neglect" with "plaster falling constantly in some wards, paint peeling off the walls in huge blobs, and floors rotting steadily."[24] The publication of this report can only have added to the tension around the need for new facilities to be built for Manhattan State Hospital, either on Ward's Island or elsewhere.

As the pressure mounted, behind the scenes, it all came down to Robert Moses. As late as 1944, he stated in a letter his "hope that the State postwar program for the Department of Mental Hygiene will include provision for the present Ward's Island inmates at other hospitals in the suburbs," but by 1945 he seems to have tired of the issue and agreed to a meeting with Frederick MacCurdy, New York State Commissioner of Mental Hygiene. A backroom deal appears to have been made, and in a letter dated June 28, 1945, Moses stated that he had been presented with "an entirely satisfactory compromise plan for Ward's Island": "They are going to rebuild the hospital on the land they retain including an entirely new power plant. It will ultimately have a capacity of 3,000 patients. It leaves us with sufficient land for an adequate park."[25] The agreement eventually led to legislation and a new funding allotment, and by 1946 the hospital's annual report glowed that "this year we can look forward to the future with more than hope. By legislative enactment, the state has been allocated the northwest portion of Ward's Island. There will be sufficient terrain on which to erect multistoried buildings . . . [that] will accommodate enough beds to permit sufficient time for observation of the large numbers received at this institution." Manhattan State Hospital had been granted a new lease on life.

4

THE *FRENCH CONNECTION* CONNECTION

By the early 1950s, a new vision of Ward's Island—as the site of *both* a state psychiatric hospital (with new, modern facilities) and park space to provide recreational opportunities for the residents of East Harlem—had come into focus. Following the arrangement made in 1945 between Parks Commissioner Robert Moses and Mental Hygiene Commissioner Frederick MacCurdy, in 1952 the New York state legislature and governor signed a bill giving the state a fifty-year lease on a portion of the island to be used for Manhattan State Hospital.[1] Funding was also provided for the construction of three modern "skyscraper" buildings to house up to three thousand patients within the hospital.[2] In 1955 U.S. president Dwight Eisenhower and New York governor John Dewey visited the island to lay the cornerstone for the first new building, and hospital reports from that period reflect a sense of pride and anticipation regarding the impending modernization of the facilities.[3] As will be discussed shortly, the modernization of the hospital's physical plant coincided with a revolution in the treatment of the symptoms of serious mental illnesses, facilitating a pervasive optimism within the hospital community.

Concurrent with the finalization of plans for the development of the state hospital grounds, progress was made toward the development of 122 acres of Ward's Island as an active recreation space, with a vision of picnic areas, play areas, and parking for five hundred cars. An important step was the construction of a long-promised footbridge to enable residents of Manhattan's East Harlem to access the island's park space. Constructed at the cost of roughly two million dollars and opened in 1951 with much fanfare, the 956-foot-long footbridge spanned from 103rd Street directly to Ward's Island (see figure 4.1); it was touted as providing "a long-sought and much needed neighborhood improvement" for Harlem's predominantly low-income residents.[4] Its opening was announced with a ribbon-cutting ceremony attended by both Mayor Vincent Impellitteri and Commissioner Moses, who led a parade of "scampering" children across the bridge span, to enjoy the island's amenities, including two playgrounds, two baseball fields, two softball fields, open play fields, and a "shorefront promenade." In characteristic fashion, Moses also used the occasion as an opportunity to attack "critics,

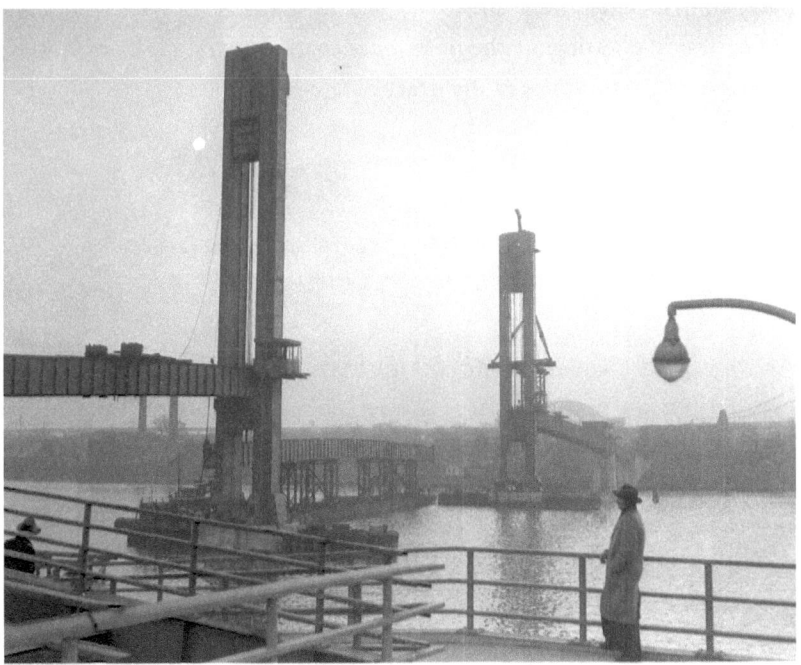

FIGURE 4.1 The Ward's Island footbridge under construction in 1950.

Source: *New York Daily News*.

detractors, smart-alecks and planning experts" who had decried his efforts to turn Ward's Island into a park.[5]

A detail that was rarely mentioned in glowing reports at the time, however, was that the footbridge lay on the other side of the recently constructed Harlem River Drive, so that anyone seeking to traverse it would need to take an additional highway overpass to reach it. The overpass, in turn, was located four long blocks (roughly three-quarters of a mile) from the nearest subway stop on Lexington Avenue. Possibly as a result, three years after its opening, published accounts indicate that the island's recreational facilities were significantly underused. One 1954 *New York Times* article noted that the crowds were so sparse that a concession stand was closed for lack of business; another observed that fewer than a thousand people visited the park on a summer Sunday.[6] While praising the beauty of the island's facilities, the articles implied that the distance that had to be walked to get to and then cross the footbridge likely contributed to their underuse. An additional factor not mentioned, but certainly plausible, is the possibility that potential park-goers were deterred by the presence of the nearby state hospital.

A TREATMENT REVOLUTION AT MANHATTAN STATE HOSPITAL

As we saw in chapters 2 and 3, Manhattan State Hospital gradually evolved from offering services in the tradition of "moral treatment" (engaging patients in structured activity such as maintaining the hospital grounds, including farmland) to providing somatic-based treatments such as insulin and electric shock, pharmacologic agents, and even psychosurgery. We also saw how a tremendous influx of elderly patients with dementias and stroke-related conditions contributed to a reduced emphasis on treatments that included physical activity. In the mid-1950s, the hospital's focus on somatic-based treatments evolved further following a French pharmacologic "revolution"—the introduction of the drug chlorpromazine, commercial name Thorazine, the first of a class of drugs that came to be known as antipsychotic medications, used as a treatment for psychosis to this day.[7]

Chlorpromazine, a chemical first synthesized by the French chemist Paul Charpentier in 1951, was investigated as a possible anesthetic by the French surgeon Henri Laborit, who noticed that patients who were administered the drug became passive and disinterested but did not lose consciousness. Laborit thought that the passive, disinterested state it induced might be useful in managing psychosis. In 1952 he convinced colleagues at Paris's St. Anne's Hospital to administer the agent to a patient experiencing acute psychosis and noted that it had an immediate calming effect. Following the publication of a case report on this initial administration, additional research was conducted and findings published. By 1954 the potential effectiveness of chlorpromazine was recognized around the world, and the drug was being manufactured by the U.S. pharmaceutical company Smith, Kline and French (now GlaxoSmithKline).

Annual reports indicate that chlorpromazine was first used in the hospital in September 1954 with a group of eight hundred "perpetually disturbed" patients. Although "not all patients... responded so well," overall "the transformation in the disturbed ward picture has been most striking."[8] Use of the drug and related agents progressed rapidly between 1955 and 1960, with reports indicating that of the hospital's roughly 3,500 patients, about 1,100 received the agent in 1958, 1,700 in 1959, and 1,900 in 1960.

Beyond the widespread administration of chlorpromazine, the late 1950s were years of great change and optimism for the hospital. After nearly a hundred years of annual reports continuously lamenting overcrowding, dilapidated structures, and understaffing, the reports of 1957–1961 were the most glowing and optimistic ones I have read, suggesting that the hospital had entered something of a "golden age," at least from the perspective of its administrators. In 1958 the first of the three new promised "skyscrapers" opened, a twenty-one-story structure known as the Medico-Surgical Building (now the Dunlap Building). Coinciding with the opening of the structure, the hospital elected to implement an "open hospital" approach, in which patients were free to move about the building, going to places like the "community store" and using the phone. Individual and group psychotherapy sessions were also offered to a larger number of patients than previously by a group of ten psychiatrists with a specific interest in these approaches; a total of 375 patients received psychotherapy in 1958. The 1958 annual report noted that "the patients highly appreciated this individual attention." There was also an increased emphasis on discharge from the hospital, with roughly eight hundred patients living in the community while still considered patients at the hospital (a step toward hospital discharge previously known as parole but now called convalescent care). The 1957 report specifically linked an increase in discharges from the hospital to the psychotropic revolution, noting that "since the chlorpromazine venture, so many more patients left the hospital that it became expedient for this institution to establish its own clinic independent of the metropolitan group."[9] Annual reports indicate a decrease in the Manhattan State Hospital census, which declined from roughly 3,600 in 1956 to 3,200 in 1960 (a decrease of about 11 percent). This paralleled a broader decrease in the state hospital system, described in the 1957 statewide report.

There was even a focus on assisting patients with seeking employment before their transfer to convalescent care. Members of the larger community seemed interested in helping patients and offering resources: the celebrity broadcaster Hugh Downs set up a hospital radio broadcasting station, and the New York Yankees baseball team offered tickets to interested patients to attend home games at nearby Yankee Stadium in the Bronx. The second two new buildings (now called Meyer and Kirby) opened in 1959 and 1960 to further fanfare. Appearing satisfied that his work was done, the director John Travis retired in 1960. By 1961 lobotomy and insulin-coma therapies had been officially discontinued, and it was noted that "they were not missed." There is a sense from reports that patients could come to the hospital, receive effective treatment in a comfortable setting, and have a reasonable chance of being discharged back into the community.

Supporting the view that attitudes within the hospital had changed, an academic publication from 1963, authored by the hospital psychiatrist Dr. Herman Denber, describes the development of the hospital's eighty-five-bed "research unit" in the late 1950s.[10] Denber discussed the creation of an open hospital policy in 1957 that went further than what is described in the annual reports, stating that "patients were encouraged to go to the city where they could either see shows, take walks, visit museums, or the like" and that "a very liberal policy was followed regarding home visits." In addition to pharmacologic treatment, there were regular group psychotherapy meetings and discussions between staff and patients. Though not presenting any specific findings, Denber reported that patients "responded rapidly to the warm, accepting and friendly environment." He also acknowledged challenges, however, conceding that there was considerable resistance to the open hospital policy: nursing staff "were bewildered by the scope and meaning of the new program, for it was completely antithetical to what they had been taught and what had been common hospital practice since its opening." Other units in the hospital did not follow the same philosophy, suggesting that the hospital administration was ambivalent about the "liberal" approach being followed in the research unit. Although the article expressed optimism about the possibility of culture change within the mental health system, it made it clear that it was an uphill battle.

Broader systemic changes operating in the late 1950s and early 1960s influenced what was happening at Manhattan State Hospital and the optimistic climate within it. In 1954 New York State passed the Community Mental Health Services Act, which allocated funding to community-based care mechanisms, including "outpatient psychiatric clinics" and "inpatient psychiatric services in general hospitals."[11] An article from 1957 suggests that the move toward community-based care came not from the development of chlorpromazine but from a concern with the constantly rising population in the state hospital system (more than ninety thousand statewide in 1954, double what it had been twenty-five years earlier, an increase that far exceeded population growth) and from a postwar interest in the prevention of mental disorder.[12] The Community Mental Health Services Act provided a funding mechanism that facilitated the opening of the community convalescent care clinic described in the hospital's annual report, as well as other community-based services to which Manhattan State Hospital patients could be referred upon discharge. Spending for community-based services within New York City nearly doubled within two years, going from nine million dollars in 1954 to $15.5 million in 1956.

On a national level, the belief that, with the help of the newly developed medications, people diagnosed with mental illness could successfully live in the community was becoming increasingly prominent. As the historian Gerald Grob has documented in *The Mad Among Us*, his landmark historical study of U.S. mental health service system, the move toward community reentry was "in the air" at this time, and chlorpromazine only reinforced this approach.[13] The 1948 publication of Albert Deutsch's *The Shame of the States*, documenting terrible conditions at state psychiatric hospitals around the country (including Manhattan State Hospital, as discussed in the previous chapter), contributed to the widespread opinion that a move away from state hospitals was needed.[14] Efforts to move toward community-based care gained momentum with the 1961 publication of *Action for Mental Health* by the Joint Commission on Mental Illness and Health, a group of experts appointed by President Eisenhower, who recommended that community-based services for people with mental illnesses be substantially increased.[15] These forces not only molded the views and sensibilities of practitioners and administrators like Dr. Denber but also directly affected the availability of resources to transition patients out of the hospital and provide them with time-intensive treatments such as psychotherapy.

DETERIORATION OF THE HOSPITAL IN THE 1970s

What happened at Manhattan State Hospital in the 1960s and 1970s? Sadly, official hospital reports disappear from the public record after 1961, so I am unable to determine the views of hospital administrators about conditions following the "golden age" evident in the reports from 1957 to 1961.[16] However, media reports from the 1970s paint a very negative picture of the treatment environment in the hospital, indicating that the "golden age" had come to an end sometime in the 1960s. A *New York*

Times article from 1974 suggested that criminal acts, including robbery, assault, and rape, were rampant in the hospital, leading to "pervasive fear," and alleged that "inadequate security" had allowed this to occur.[17] Contrary to popular assumptions about mental illness and criminality, however, these criminal acts were generally perpetrated not *by* patients but rather *against* them, by community members who gained entry by making copies of ward keys. Although hospital administrators downplayed the frequency of these incidents, the article indicated that they were calling for an end to the open hospital policy and the installation of a security gate separating the hospital from the larger Ward's Island Park. Besides alleging an atmosphere of fear, the article described the atmosphere as "depressing," reporting that "in day rooms, the television plays and patients sometimes curl up and sleep in chairs" and quoting from a patient's poem, "they play with their hands here for hours / afloat on fingers of boredom." These vignettes paint a poignant picture of inactivity at the hospital, suggesting a deterioration in the enthusiastic and hopeful atmosphere portrayed in the reports from 1957 to 1961.

Larger societal trends, in New York City and nationally, likely affected the climate within and around Manhattan State Hospital during the 1960s and early 1970s. The psychologist Steven Pinker has characterized the cultural changes during this period as a "de-civilizing" process that resulted from the elevation of youthful impulsiveness over self-control and societal connectedness (though he also recognized the importance of the many rights movements of the 1960s in reducing targeted violence toward women, African Americans, and gay and lesbian individuals).[18] I would add that the Vietnam War, which many people considered to be unjust, the drafting of young men to serve in it, and the assassinations of admired leaders including President Kennedy and Martin Luther King Jr. all contributed to a sense of alienation and anger among young people. Regardless of the cause, the pattern is clear. As recorded by the FBI, between 1965 and 1975 rates of violent crime in New York State increased almost threefold, from 325 to 856 per 100,000 (for context, the rate was down to 350 per 100,000 in 2018).[19] The murder of Kitty Genovese in 1964 in Queens (where it was reported that neighbors heard her cries but declined to intervene) was viewed as a bellwether event in public concern about violent crime, especially in New York City. Although it is now generally agreed that the reporting of neighbor inaction in the Kitty Genovese incident was seriously flawed, the way the event captured the public imagination cannot be denied.

Simultaneously, police departments in major cities, including New York, are believed to have been engaged (whether by design or de facto) in a policy of "benign neglect" in low-income communities of color, to which Ward's Island—technically part of the then predominantly Hispanic East Harlem—was connected. The term, coined in 1970 by Daniel Patrick Moynihan (an adviser to President Richard Nixon and later a U.S. senator), implied that failing to engage in law enforcement in low-income communities might somehow be beneficial to these communities. In *The Savage City*, T. J. English discusses how, parallel to this neglect, police corruption, with officers turning a blind eye to activities such as gambling, drug dealing, and prostitution in exchange for cash bribes, was rampant in Harlem at the time, leading to a general feeling of distrust in social systems among community members.[20] At the same time, social norms had begun to change, and the availability and use of illegal drugs became exponentially greater, particularly among young people. Capturing the scale of this growth are findings from a report by researchers at the National Institute of Drug Abuse, which estimated that the number of annual marijuana "initiates" in the United States grew twenty-fold between 1962 and 1973, while the number of annual cocaine "initiates" grew nearly seventy-fold during the same time period.[21]

All of these social forces no doubt affected the frequency and nature of the interactions between the Harlem community and the residents of Manhattan State Hospital, who had only recently been connected to each other via footbridge and public bus. Hospital patients residing on an open ward or on convalescent care status were free to enter the community and could meet and develop friendships and other relationships with community members; given some of the trends of the time, it is plausible that in some of these interactions, community members involved in crime or substance use might seek to exploit the patients. Many patients, having lived in a controlled setting for so long, might have lacked the "street smarts" to differentiate between a genuine and an ill-intentioned social interaction. By the mid-1960s, the corner of 125th Street and Lexington Avenue—the terminus of the island's only public transportation connection to Manhattan—had developed enough of a reputation as a location for drug selling that it was mentioned in a song about buying heroin by the Velvet Underground, the transgressive New York band led by Lou Reed.[22] Clearly there were ample opportunities for patients traveling into the community to be approached by drug sellers or users. As the mental health system would learn in a few years (see chapter 5), people with serious mental health conditions might be particularly sensitive to these now readily available substances, potentially leading to a cascade of negative effects.

Another social force that may have affected the treatment climate within Manhattan State Hospital is what Jonathan Metzl characterized as the increased "racialization" of schizophrenia in the United States in the late 1960s.[23] Metzl discusses how, with the publication in 1968 of the diagnostic guide known as the DSM-II, schizophrenia became increasingly equated with a presumed "hostile and aggressive" stance that was associated with that of many Black men's participation in the civil rights protests of the time. For example, he discusses how psychiatry came to brand beliefs in the pervasive impact of racism as "paranoid delusions." This pattern, as part of the zeitgeist of the late 1960s and early 1970s, may have led service providers to take an increasingly hostile stance toward patients whom they may have begun to view with fear rather than compassion. Racial discrimination in treatment would operate independently and in addition to the causal role that racial discrimination appears to play in leading to psychotic experiences (discussed in chapter 3), but would be expected to have a negative impact on outcomes among those who had already been diagnosed.

At the same time as these social forces were affecting the safety climate within Manhattan State Hospital, New York State was expecting the hospital to do more with less. In the early 1970s the United States experienced a period of economic stagnation (both rising inflation and rising unemployment), triggered in part by the 1973 oil crisis, which affected tax revenues and public spending.[24] In 1976 funding for state hospitals was cut in the New York State budget.[25] Yet the hospital was held liable for the impact of the cuts when, in 1977, New York State Comptroller Arthur Levitt published a report based on investigations of Manhattan State Hospital and two other hospitals, alleging "severe fiscal mismanagement, a shortage of linen . . . and poor security." The hospital's response to the report noted that the patient population of the hospital had increased by 20 percent during this time period because of the transfer of patients from the Pilgrim State Hospital on Long Island—ironically the hospital that large numbers of patients from Manhattan State Hospital had been transferred *to* in the 1930s.[26]

EFFORTS TO IMPROVE HOSPITAL CONDITIONS

In his response to the state comptroller's report, the hospital's newly appointed director, Dr. Gabriel Koz, did not deny its allegations but expressed high hopes for the hospital, stating "we deal with people from Manhattan who are the most sick and the most needy, so they should get the best care, not the worst." He further noted that he wished to make use of the beautiful setting to further the rehabilitative aims of the hospital: "There should be parks and gardens. There should be a sculpture garden out there. There could be jogging tracks." Although there are no reports of Dr. Koz succeeding in opening jogging tracks on Ward's Island, he did succeed in opening a sculpture garden on the island's grounds, which received some media coverage.[27] A 1981 review of the sculpture garden in the local arts-oriented magazine *Soho News* was positive, but it noted the relative inaccessibility of the island and the fact that there were no places to eat on it ("pack your own lunch and take a thermos").[28] Koz also engaged art students from Brooklyn's Pratt Institute in a project to beautify the interior of the hospital, which received a commendation from the American Psychiatric Association's Community and State Hospital Division for "transforming a formerly drab institution into an aesthetic human environment."[29]

A journal article written by Dr. Koz in 1979 provides a detailed picture of what was now being called the Manhattan Psychiatric Center and how hard it was for it to accomplish what it was being tasked with.[30] The capacity of the hospital had been reduced to 1,500 beds, less than half of what it was in 1961, indicating that significant numbers of patients had either been discharged or passed away and their slots not refilled (a newspaper article from 1980 reported that the actual hospital census at that time was 1,315).[31] This decrease was to be expected, given the advent of the policy that became known as deinstitutionalization, which gained momentum after the federal Community Mental Health Center Act in 1963, as well the development of nursing homes as an alternate location for elderly patients with dementia. Between 1962 and 1972, there was a national decrease in the number of elderly in state psychiatric hospitals of roughly 50 percent, mostly as a result of transfers to nursing homes.[32] Between 1955 and 1980, there was a roughly 75 percent decrease in total patient population in state hospitals nationally. Published analyses of trends in the New York State hospital population indicate a decline of 72 percent during that period, with the decline occurring mostly before 1972 and slowing thereafter.[33] Therefore, it is likely that a large proportion of Manhattan State Hospital's population reduction came from both discharges to the community and transfers to nursing care.

Despite the declining census, Dr. Koz argued that the hospital was underfunded, noting that the budget provided was sixty dollars per patient per day ($268 in 2023 dollars), considerably more than in the late 1800s and early 1900s but roughly five to ten times less than is spent today.[34] He characterized this as much lower than what he had been allocated in a municipal hospital where he had previously worked, and much less than what was needed. He also noted difficulties in staffing, with only one psychiatrist available for each ward of forty patients and eight registered nurses for a four-ward unit of 150 patients (meaning only about one registered nurse per shift for 150 patients, given the need to fill all the days of the week and overnight shifts). Although Dr. Koz celebrated the changes since 1961 that had brought about a significant reduction in the "warehousing" of patients, he also emphasized that, as a result of underfunding and an entrenched civil service mentality, "the standards of care . . . are still far from acceptable." Emphasizing the disjoint between high need and the level of resources that had always been part of the hospital's conundrum, he echoed the words of Dr. Alexander MacDonald roughly a hundred years earlier, concluding that "if one were asked to design a very bad system of psychiatric care for those patients who need care the most, the result would be what we now have in the state of New York."[35]

A GROWTH IN NEW INSTITUTIONAL POPULATIONS

Even as the patient population at Manhattan State Hospital was declining, the late 1960s and early 1970s saw the introduction of new institutions to Ward's Island for the first time since the late 1800s. The allure of Ward's Island as the location for institutions that could be sited without community opposition appeared to remain strong. In 1965 newly elected New York governor Nelson Rockefeller pledged funding to build a two-hundred-bed hospital devoted to the treatment of children with psychiatric problems on the island, not far from the grounds of Manhattan State Hospital.[36] The new hospital, which became known as Manhattan Children's Psychiatric Center, did not open until approximately 1971.[37] Although no information is available on the characteristics of the children served in the 1970s, a report published in 1987 (based on a visit conducted in 1985) indicated that the center served eighty inpatients and fifty-five outpatients, so it is unlikely that the two-hundred-bed capacity was ever reached.[38] A report published in 1990 (based on data collected in the 1980s) indicates that the population served was between the ages of five and thirteen, predominantly male (88 percent), and overwhelmingly Black or Hispanic (93 percent). They were diagnosed with conditions such as conduct disorder and ADHD and were mainly offered structured day treatment, in which children attended a series of groups throughout the day.[39]

A related institution emerged, with significantly less planning, when of one of the buildings that had been part of Manhattan State Hospital before the construction of the three new buildings (the Keener Building, figure 4.2), was rapidly called into service in 1973 to house sixty-three children with severe intellectual disabilities.[40] The abrupt move was a consequence of an infamous exposé of conditions at the Willowbrook State School in Staten Island (conducted by a brash young reporter, Geraldo Rivera), which led the state to transfer children from Willowbrook to new facilities.[41] When an additional 125 children were transferred to Keener in 1974 from a community-based setting that had experienced a gas leak, the remoteness of Ward's Island was discussed as a major drawback. An article quoted one advocate who said "the children are in exile" because it was so hard for family members to reach the island and another who pointed out that the young people who had learned to go to stores independently could no longer do so: "Where can they go to a store . . . on this island?"[42] Although the children who had been moved due to the gas leak were able to return after about a month, the children originally moved from Willowbrook remained at Keener for another three years, no less in exile.[43]

A third new institution opened in 1971 when one of the former Manhattan State Hospital buildings was rented to the relatively new substance use treatment program, Odyssey House. The building, named after early hospital superintendent William Mabon, now dubbed itself the "mothers and babies of narcotics" (MABON) building; it was used to house the Parent's Program, a twelve- to eighteen-month residential

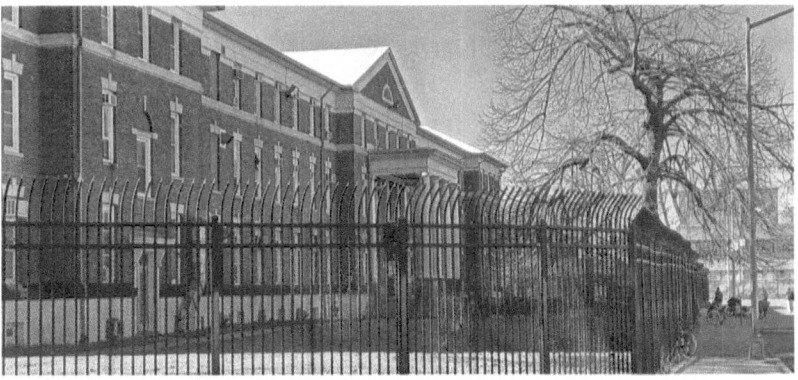

FIGURE 4.2 The Keener Building, November 23, 2023.

Source: Photo by author.

substance use treatment program for expectant mothers and mothers of children under five (the mothers were allowed to reside with their young children).[44] Odyssey House, founded by the psychiatrist Dr. Judianne Densen-Gerber, was part of a new brand of treatment programs known as "therapeutic communities" that had started cropping up in the wake of the dramatic increase in substance use and abuse discussed previously. These programs required total abstinence and placed an emphasis on rules and order. In the case of Odyssey House, there does not appear to have been much concern about the remoteness of the island, as residents were expected to remain inside the setting for the duration of their stay. An Odyssey House program remains on Ward's Island to this day (see chapter 6).

FROM PARKLAND TO CRIMINAL HAVEN?

Ward's Island Park remained open throughout the growth in institutions described here, but did it draw the crowds that were envisioned by Robert Moses? It might be reasonable to expect that, after being on the scene for several years, word would get out and Ward's Island would achieve its promise as a park for New York City's residents, but evidence does not support that this occurred. After reporting that the park was underutilized in the early 1950s, in 1963 the *New York Times* reported that it was neglected and littered with "widespread debris," indicating a complete lack of park department attention.[45] By the 1960s, despite investing resources to create a landfill connection between Ward's and Randall's Islands, Moses himself seems to have conceded that the island would not become a major recreational destination for New Yorkers.[46] By the early 1970s its reputation had deteriorated further, and it was viewed as a location where criminals could operate freely without concern of detection. This was reflected in the Academy Award–winning police drama *The French Connection*, which featured the island as the wild and lawless location of a major heroin distribution hideout. A pivotal scene in which New York City police engage in a shootout with the heroin distribution leaders was filmed on the island near the imposing columns of the Hell Gate Bridge (see figure 4.3). The filming took place shortly after my family and I had moved to the island, and, though I was quite young, I recall my father being excited to view the filming of the pivotal scene from the sidelines.

Despite the sensationalized picture painted by *The French Connection* and reflected in some media reports, I do not have any memories of living in fear on Ward's Island in the 1970s. My brother and our small number of friends (the children of other employees who lived on the island) played freely and largely unsupervised outside. My main memory is of its being quiet and empty (see figure 4.4), with the main safety concern being roving packs of wild dogs that had somehow found a home on the island. On the night of July 13, 1977, when New York City experienced a total loss of electric power and other parts of the city experienced looting and other forms of chaos, I just remember being able to see a sky full of stars, something I had never seen before. I recently asked my

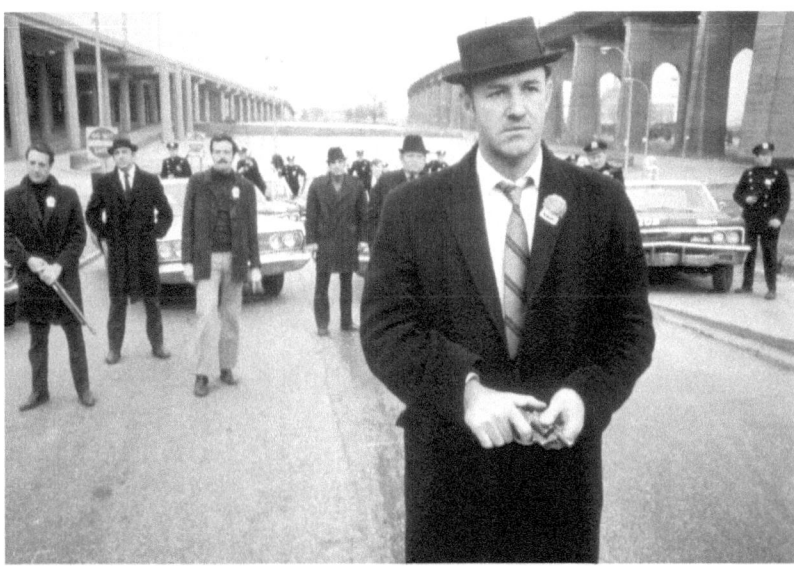

FIGURE 4.3 Police officers preparing to enter Ward's Island to confront drug dealers in *The French Connection*.

Source: Getty Images.

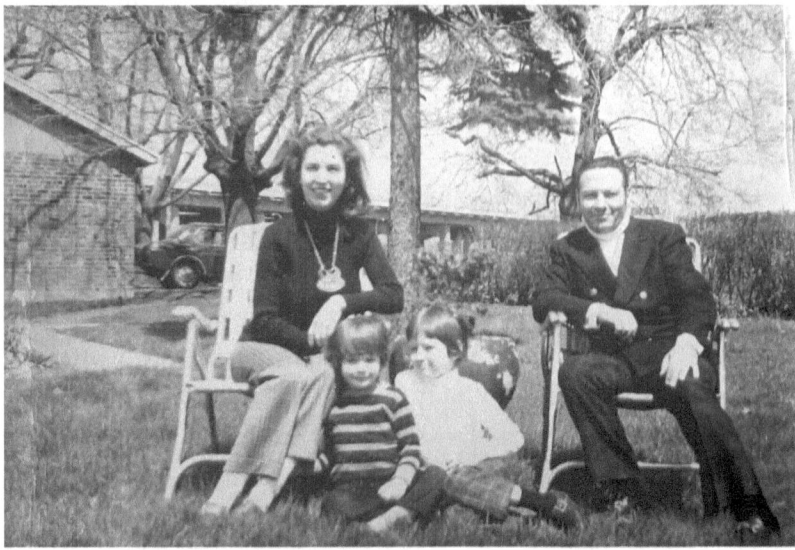

FIGURE 4.4 Yanos family photo on Ward's Island, 1970s.

Source: Photo by Theodore Yanos.

mother about her memories, and she corroborated that the island was a "nice, quiet" place to live. However, our memories *do* support the idea that Ward's Island was not frequented by the larger New York community. When I told other children in my Manhattan parochial school where I lived, they almost never knew where it was nor had they ever visited it. My mother corroborated that this was her experience with adults as well. Ward's Island was definitely off the beaten track, much better known as the location of institutions than as a place of recreation or relaxation. City leaders were undoubtedly aware of this; Ward's Island's role as a place of exile for urban outcasts was about to expand.

5

"IN ACCORDANCE WITH THE STANDARDS"

As the 1970s came to an end and Edward Koch took over as New York City's mayor, it became evident to city residents that a new and different problem was beginning to manifest itself: increasing numbers of people without a home (soon to be referred to as "the homeless"). This problem would soon reach a crisis point and inaugurate a new era in the history of Ward's Island's as a haven for the dumping of New York's most marginalized.

As described by medical anthropologist Kim Hopper and others, homelessness had existed throughout New York City's history, but it tended to increase dramatically during times of widespread economic distress, such as the Great Depression, when shantytowns were built in city parks by those who had recently lost their homes.[1] The city's first public shelter was founded around the turn of the twentieth century on a barge located at the foot of East Twenty-Sixth Street, near Bellevue Hospital. The city later established a municipal shelter in a building on East Twenty-Fifth Street; it moved to East Third Street and the Bowery (in what is now known as the East Village) in the late 1940s.[2] This shelter could accommodate up to six hundred men per night, although its bed capacity was far below this, and many men slept on the floor during cold nights. The Bowery was also home to a number of inexpensive lodging houses that the city provided vouchers for men to stay in, which relieved overcrowding at the shelter (sources note that the city would provide roughly a thousand vouchers on typical days and as many as 1,500 during the winter).[3]

In the late 1970s, as the city phased out the voucher program, it became evident that the Bowery Municipal Shelter could no longer accommodate the number of people seeking its services, leading greater numbers to sleep in the lobby or outside on the street.[4] At the same time, the nature of those presenting for shelter was changing. Previously, the typical person coming to the municipal shelter fit the stereotype of a "hobo"—an older white male with alcohol problems. However, in the late 1970s, those presenting were increasingly likely to be younger, be Black or Hispanic, and appear to have a mental illness or report a history of psychiatric treatment. (An awareness that women were also susceptible to homelessness did not emerge until the 1980s.) In 1978 two psychiatrists described the Bowery as a "psychiatric dumping ground," providing case descriptions of a number of young men (mostly of color) who were presenting with psychiatric problems at the municipal shelter.[5] Dr. Hopper, who conducted ethnographic fieldwork on the Bowery around that time, observed that the presence of people with psychiatric problems on the Bowery was "impossible to miss."[6]

By the 1980s it was evident that the problem of homelessness was getting worse, and a group of public-interest lawyers affiliated with the Legal Aid Society, including Robert Hayes and Wendy Addis (who would later form the Coalition for the Homeless), filed a class-action suit against both New York City and New York State. The suit argued that Article XVII of the New York State Constitution, which declares that "the aid, care and support of the needy are public concerns and shall be provided by the state" provided a right to shelter and that the city and state therefore had a responsibility to expand the range of shelter options for men without homes. State judge Andrew Tyler reviewed the case and ordered that New York City and State immediately provide 750 additional beds to house homeless men during the winter.[7]

In a scramble to identify suitable locations that would not arouse community opposition, the newly elected mayor, Edward Koch, selected the Keener Building on Ward's Island, which (as we saw in chapter 4) had been used to house intellectually disabled children from Willowbrook but had been vacated in 1977. In his autobiography, Dr. Gabriel Koz, then the director of the Manhattan Psychiatric Center, discusses being invited to a clandestine meeting at City Hall with Mayor Koch to discuss the feasibility of Keener's serving as a shelter location.[8] Although the Legal Aid lawyers initially opposed the Keener location, they ultimately agreed to it because many of the affected men indicated that it would be acceptable. Speaking in retrospect, Robert Hayes stated:

> We, young idealists, thought this was abhorrent: to create a shelter on the grounds of a psychiatric institution, on an island in the middle of the East River, shoving humanity out of sight. And we were ready to try to block that, arguing that the operation was basically a sham: the building was inaccessible, and nobody would go there. But talking to some homeless individuals then living at the Bowery, I learned that those sheltered at the Keener Building were relieved to get away from the pressure and the stress of the hard-living conditions of the Lower East Side. They were welcoming the Keener Building as a refuge.[9]

Although Dr. Koz did not oppose the opening of the shelter, there was some opposition from members of the Manhattan Psychiatric Center and Manhattan Children's Psychiatric Center communities, who warned that it would create a "dangerous and perilous" situation for hospital patients. However, the urgency of the situation in the middle of winter overrode their protests.[10] By early January, Keener was already being used to house roughly 180 men when it was visited by Mayor Koch, who stated "it's not exactly a palace, but it's nice" (see figure 5.1).[11] A resident quoted in an article after the mayor's visit concurred, stating, "It's sort of like a resort here, much nicer than the Men's Shelter."[12]

Initially, the Keener shelter was meant to be a temporary solution to increased homelessness during the winter, and it was planned to be discontinued by the end of May. However, the planned closure of Keener did not occur, and by the following winter 510 men were staying there, well over the official bed capacity of 242.[13] Shortly thereafter, the city and state agreed to build a four-hundred-bed addition to the Keener shelter,

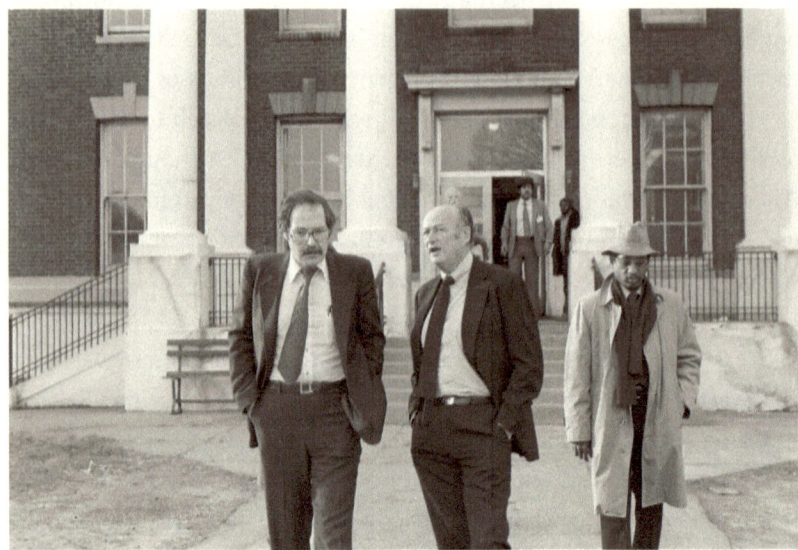

FIGURE 5.1 Mayor Edward Koch outside the Keener Building in 1980.

Source: New York City Municipal Archives.

which was already being described as "overcrowded, filthy and overrun by vermin," a far cry from how it had been initially assessed.[14] The expansion proceeded despite further opposition from a group representing Manhattan Children's Psychiatric Center, who complained that shelter residents upset children by using vulgar language on the city bus.[15] By August 1981, an official legal decision was made that became known as the Callahan Consent Decree, after Robert Callahan, a Korean War veteran, who was the lead plaintiff in the case brought by the Legal Aid attorneys. The Keener shelter was specifically named in the consent decree as one of three facilities to be operated in accordance with certain specific standards, including:

- a bed of a minimum thirty inches in width,
- a clean, comfortable, well-constructed mattress,
- and two clean sheets, a clean blanket, a clean pillow case, a clean towel, and soap and toilet tissue.[16]

The Callahan Consent Decree established New York City's "right to shelter," which remains in effect to this day (although city government has recently tried to argue that it applies only to specific groups of "citizens").[17]

CAUSES OF THE PROBLEM

In the immediate aftermath of the opening of Keener and the Callahan Consent Decree, there was a back-and-forth between the city and the state governments about what had happened, who was at fault, and who should bear fiscal responsibility going forward. The city, noting that increasing numbers of individuals presenting for services appeared to be "mentally ill," blamed the state for a "failure to plan and support programs to help [formerly hospitalized] individuals cope with life on the outside" in lieu of deinstitutionalization.[18] The state, in turn, lashed out at the city for changes in housing policy that had led to a dramatic reduction in the stock of affordable housing for unemployed persons and others living at the margins, specifically by giving tax incentives to owners of single-room-occupancy hotels to convert them to more expensive dwellings.[19] Single-room-occupancy hotels (SROs) had long served as the city's least expensive housing choice for single adults, including immigrant men, such as my father when he returned to New York in the late 1940s after living in Greece, and many others when they first arrived as immigrants without their families.

Who was right? In the short term, the data largely supported the state's argument. Although it was true, as we saw in chapter 4, that the state hospital population in New York had declined by more than 70 percent between 1955 and 1980, the bulk of the decrease had been completed by 1972—a full five years before the increase in homelessness and the apparent presence of "former mental patients" among their ranks had been noted. If the state had "dumped" people onto the streets, why had they not appeared until more than twenty years after the "dumping" had started? Further supporting the state's argument was evidence that the conversion of SROs, which began in the early 1960s, had accelerated dramatically in the late 1970s. Analyses indicate that roughly one hundred thousand SRO units were lost between 1960 and 1978, and more than ten thousand between 1975 and 1979 alone.[20] SROs were one of the only types of housing that former hospital residents living on public benefits such as Supplemental Security Income ($177.80 per month in 1977) could afford at a time when the average monthly rent in New York City was more than three hundred dollars.[21] The decline in SRO units, incentivized by New York City tax policy, was part of a larger trend of "gentrification" that would only accelerate in the 1980s, when average rents would rise to $1,700 per month.[22] Simultaneously, other housing was lost to "abandonment," at a rate of 31,000 units per year between 1970 and 1981, as landlords decided to walk away from distressed properties in less affluent areas.[23] As Dr. Hopper noted in 1988, "individual failures to procure stable housing thus have their roots in larger, system-wide developments. . . . The special plight of the mentally disabled must be placed within this overall context of sharpened competition for an increasingly scarce and costly commodity." Echoing this are the findings from a recent exhaustive study by policy analysts Gregg Colburn and Clayton Page Aldern of variations in the rates of homelessness on a national level. Likening the interaction between individual and structural factors to a game of musical chairs, they conclude: "Regional variation in rates of homelessness can be explained by the costs and availability of housing . . . people with health and economic vulnerabilities live in every city . . . the difference is the location context in which they live."[24] In New York City in the late 1970s, people with serious mental illnesses who had both health and economic vulnerability were increasingly likely to wind up without a chair when the music stopped.

In the longer term, however, as homelessness continued to grow in 1980s, it is likely that new changes in state policy began to contribute to the overrepresentation of people with serious mental illnesses among those without a home. In 1980 the state announced that the criteria for admission to state hospitals would be made more stringent, stating that "the popular perception of the Office of Mental Health as the primary provider of mental health services is a holdover from former times."[25]

An Office of Mental Health official made it clear that state hospitals could not be used as a substitute for lack of housing: "we don't admit people who are maybe a little strange and don't have a place to live." This policy change, whatever its merits, was ill-timed, placing increased pressure on the city at a time when it was scrambling to catch up with the demand for shelter amid the market forces of gentrification that it had helped unleash. A review of formal studies conducted in the 1980s found that between 10 and 30 percent of people living in shelters or similar locations had psychiatric treatment histories (greater than what would be expected in the general population, where the prevalence of serious mental illness is generally estimated to be 5 percent).[26]

Thus, many of the newly homeless individuals with mental illnesses would have been not deinstitutionalized but never institutionalized (although a number would interact with the state hospital system for briefer stays than were typical in earlier eras). Many of the newly homeless were too young to have lived in a state hospital during the 1960s, when deinstitutionalization was in full swing. In 1981, three clinicians working within an outpatient program affiliated with a New York State hospital inaugurated awareness of this group with a report, published in a major psychiatric journal, on what they called "the young adult chronic patient."[27] They noted that this group, aged between eighteen and thirty-five, had "spent relatively little time in hospitals but . . . present[ed] persistent and frustrating problems to community caregivers in mental health and other social service systems." A high proportion of these individuals had alcohol or substance use problems—issues that had not been previously considered a major concern among people with serious mental illnesses but that had clearly increased among those who came of age in the 1960s and 1970s. Further, many had experienced homelessness, as well as come into contact with law enforcement systems for minor criminal activity. Both substance use and legal histories likely contributed to their being turned away by family members or friends, increasing their risk for homelessness. In addition to noting the need to address substance use issues, the authors noted a "crying need for residential programs" for this group to reduce homelessness.

Other evidence indicated that an increasing number of "young adult chronic patients" were being seen at state hospitals, but they were being discharged more quickly than the state hospital patients of years past. An article published in 1984 compared the ages of patients in all New York State hospitals between 1977 and 1982 and found that, though the proportion of male patients over forty-five had decreased by 27 percent, the proportion between twenty-five and thirty-four had increased by 22 percent.[28] They concluded that "the nature of the state psychiatric centers is changing, with declining numbers of older patients and growing numbers of younger patients who have markedly different programmatic needs."

At the same time as these young adults were being admitted to state hospitals and discharged after symptom stabilization, the state had not yet established formal mechanisms for stable housing, leading them to be discharged "back to the street." Evidence for this was provided by Dr. Hopper, who cited an internal Office of Mental Health report stating that 59 percent of all discharges from Manhattan Psychiatric Center were discharged to "unknown" living arrangements.[29] In 1982 the Coalition for the Homeless filed a suit against the state to address this situation, insisting that the state provide "minimal housing as an essential element of the adequate treatment in the least restrictive environment due" the discharged patients.[30] Ironically, the lawsuit was celebrated by the same city leaders who had resisted the coalition's lawsuits against them, though they appeared to fundamentally misunderstand its purpose, with Mayor Koch saying "I hope he has success in his suit in getting the state to reinstitutionalize those people that require it." The lawsuit resulted in the imposition of a "very strict rule" that state hospitals could not discharge patients to a shelter or the street. On the one hand, this incentivized the creation of more residential options for those discharged; on the other hand, it incentivized maintaining strict admission criteria so as to minimize the responsibility to provide housing.[31] One result of this rule was that the state eventually created "transitional living residences" (TLRs) on the campuses of its state hospitals in formerly used buildings; on Ward's Island, the state converted a former nurses' residence directly across from the hospital into such a TLR in the early 1980s.[32]

Another factor complicating homelessness was the federally initiated War on Drugs, which led to the criminalization of substance use (which was common among the "young adult chronic patients" who had come of age in the 1960s and 1970s) and increased the likelihood that people who used illegal substances would experience the disruptive force of incarceration. The War on Drugs, officially declared by President Nixon in 1971, accelerated in the 1980s with the passage of the Sentencing Reform Act of 1984 and the Anti–Drug Abuse Act of 1986. Partly as a result of these laws, the U.S. incarceration rate doubled between 1980 and 1990.[33] Incarceration affected the likelihood that one would become homeless in a myriad of ways, from the loss of housing that results from incarceration to indirect effects on family networks to the formal prohibition of people with criminal records from living in public housing. The War on Drugs was thus a factor in the disproportionate representation of people of color among people experiencing homelessness (and the facilities of Ward's Island), given that people of color are disproportionately likely to be arrested and charged for substance-related crime in the United States.[34] The federal government also decreased its investment in public housing during the 1980s, resulting in a 40 percent decrease in the number of "Section 8" housing vouchers available to New York families during this period.[35]

In summary, the causes of the marked increase in homelessness in the late 1970s and early 1980s were complex and could not be blamed on a single factor. Deinstitutionalization had increased the number of very-low-income people in need of inexpensive housing in the community, while gentrification, abandonment, and a decline in housing vouchers simultaneously removed a large amount of affordable housing from the market. The effects of gentrification became undeniable in the 1980s as homelessness began to spread to families, now by far the largest group of people supported in the shelter system. The drug culture of the 1960s and the availability of illegal drugs in low-income communities (the only ones that people with mental illnesses might be able to afford to live in) increased the likelihood that people with mental illnesses would have the opportunity to develop co-occurring substance use problems. The misguided law enforcement response to this, the War on Drugs, meant that people with co-occurring substance use problems would be increasingly likely to experience the disrupting effects of incarceration, further contributing to homelessness. This response made people of color particularly likely to be overrepresented among those without homes, which was and continues to be evident in the demographics of single adult homeless in New York City. Although the lack of city-state cooperation has been the rule, in 1990 there was a reprieve from this bickering as New York City and New York State government officials established the joint "New York–New York" agreement to establish 3,800 permanent community-based housing units for homeless adults with serious mental illness, leading to a reduction in the single adult shelter population for the first time since the homeless crisis started. In general, however, the inability of different levels of government to accept responsibility for contributing to the homelessness crisis, and a preference for finger-pointing instead, meant that there would be an element of dysfunction in efforts to address the problem, something that persists to this day.[36]

These forces would play out on a national level throughout the 1980s and 1990s, and New York City could be seen as a "canary in a coal mine" for the national homelessness crisis that has grown and persisted across the United States, with rates that vary locally depending on the availability of affordable and supported housing. In fact, although New York City initially led the way in homelessness, by 2007 New York City ranked fourth in rates of homelessness, behind Washington, DC, Boston, and San Francisco.[37]

In 2022 the Department of Housing and Urban Development estimated that there were more than 582,000 homeless persons in the United States, including roughly 233,000 (about 40 percent) who were completely unsheltered. Related to the impacts of mass incarceration resulting from the War on Drugs, Black and Hispanic Americans are dramatically overrepresented among those who are homeless, representing more than 60 percent of the homeless population overall. People with serious mental illnesses, though not the majority, are also overrepresented, in similar proportions to what was found in New York City in the 1980s, with roughly 22 percent estimated to have a serious mental illness.[38]

As the 1980s wore on, Ward's Island was increasingly called upon to serve as a haven for the "dumping" of people, both currently and recently homeless, in multiple shelters and community residences opened in former hospital buildings. By the end of the 1980s, the Keener shelter was housing 950 men, more than five times the number initially housed there when it was opened as an "emergency" shelter in 1980.[39]

THE OPENING OF KIRBY FORENSIC PSYCHIATRIC CENTER

Another development in the Ward's Island landscape during the 1980s was the conversion of one of Manhattan Psychiatric Center's three buildings (the Kirby Building) into a state Forensic Psychiatric Hospital. Forensic psychiatric hospitals occupy a particular niche in the intersection between the criminal justice and mental health systems; they are designed to house either those who have been found "not guilty by reason of insanity" (NGRI) by a court or those charged and awaiting trial but judged "not competent" to stand trial after a court-ordered evaluation. The great majority of people with mental illness who come into contact with the criminal justice system are deemed competent and are not served by forensic psychiatric centers. In New York, most people convicted of crimes who have mental illnesses receive services within the state prison system, while those charged and awaiting trial receive service at the Rikers Island Jail (I worked to help men diagnosed with mental illnesses who were housed in the general population at Rikers Island in the late 1990s). Persons judged NGRI and "not competent" are quite distinct, as the charges that could be subject to a competency evaluation could be quite minor (such as substance possession), while those that are subject to NGRI designations tend to be violent. Those in the "not competent" group also have significantly shorter lengths of stay than the

NGRI group, since the process of "competency restoration" is usually resolved within five months, whereas NGRI status tends to result in a life sentence.[40]

In the early 1980s it was determined that the number of state forensic psychiatric patients (roughly 5 percent of the overall population served by the state system) had outgrown what could be handled by Mid-Hudson Psychiatric Center, a facility located in Orange County, roughly sixty miles from New York City. Pressure to open a new forensic facility on Ward's Island increased in 1984 after two patients housed in a secure unit in the Meyer building sawed through a barred window and climbed down nine floors on an improvised rope made of bedsheets.[41] It was therefore decided to use the hospital's Kirby Building to house forensic patients and to move general psychiatric patients into available space in the other two hospital buildings. In 1985 the Kirby Forensic Psychiatric Center opened as a 150-bed forensic hospital. An analysis of the characteristics of patients in 1990 indicated that the majority (61 percent) were being held for being "not competent." About 55 percent had been homeless prior to admissions, and their demographic characteristics mirrored those of the nearby shelter population: predominantly (90 percent) male and African American (53 percent) or Hispanic (23 percent).

Although no major changes were made to the interior of the hospital as part of the conversion, a "double row of 10-foot-high fences topped with barbed wire" was added to the perimeter of the grounds (see figure 5.2).[42] The addition of the barbed-wire fence added a more menacing air to the hospital grounds, a far cry from the open hospital atmosphere that the reformers of the 1950s had envisioned.

STAGNATION AT MANHATTAN PSYCHIATRIC CENTER

Meanwhile, next door at in the Meyer and Dunlop buildings of Manhattan Psychiatric Center, after nearly being fired for not meeting the state's census reduction targets, the energetic and reform-oriented

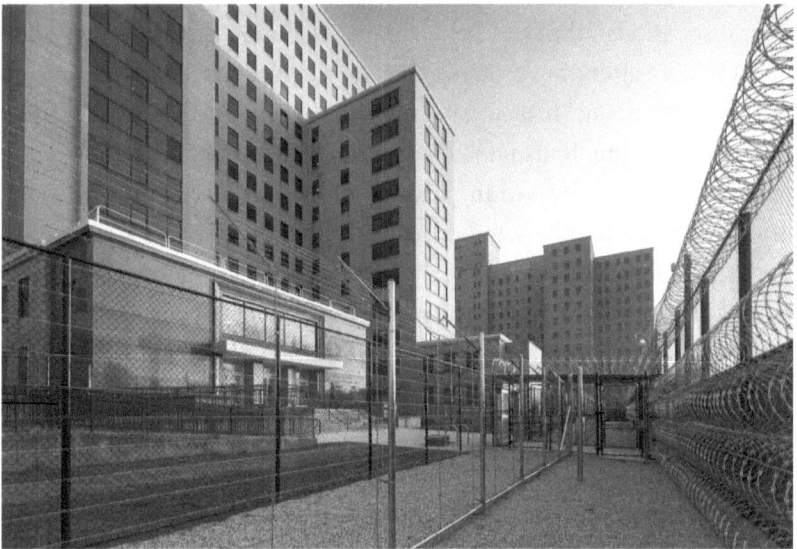

FIGURE 5.2 Barbed-wire fence around Kirby Forensic Psychiatric Center.

Source: STV Incorporated.

Dr. Koz voluntarily resigned in 1982.[43] Media reports (and Dr. Koz's retrospective account) indicate that the state hospital system moved into a period of fiscal retrenchment in the early 1980s as the costs of paying staff increased and federal support decreased.[44] An article authored by the commissioner and deputy commissioner of the state Office of Mental Health in 1985 confirmed that in the early 1980s the agency, under increasing fiscal pressure, lost its "clinical focus" and suffered an exodus of well-trained psychiatrists.[45] A 1982 article in the *New York Times* described how Pablo Martinez, a twenty-seven-year-old patient at the hospital, was beaten to death by two therapy aides (who were subsequently suspended without pay) as they struggled to restrain him, suggesting that the atmosphere had become more coercive and less therapeutic.[46]

In 1985 the New York State Commission on Quality Care for the Mentally Disabled conducted a surprise visit to Manhattan Psychiatric Center.[47] The observers noted that the hospital census at that time was 1,100, slightly lower than in the late 1970s. The report was particularly harsh in its discussion of the treatment of patients, noting that, although some patients were attending groups and engaged in art or table games, most patients were doing "little other than watching TV, sitting idly, or sleeping" and smoking. It also noted concerns with patient dress, observing that patients were dressed in pajamas and robes during the day, while others were wearing hats and coats during the day. This evidently stagnant atmosphere existed despite the fact that by this point there had been many advances in the community-based treatment of people with severe mental illnesses, approaches collectively known as psychiatric rehabilitation.[48] However, there was no evidence that a rehabilitation model was being used in the hospital.

A few years after this surprise visit, in the summer of 1989, I worked as a volunteer at Manhattan Psychiatric Center, and I can attest that, although groups were held, there was still quite a lot of watching TV, sitting idly, and sleeping going on. There was no formal use of psychiatric rehabilitation approaches such as social skills training or vocational rehabilitation that had become increasingly established by that point. It was evident to me, as I talked informally with patients in the dayroom as part of my volunteer role, that patients were hungry for more opportunities to talk and explore their experiences, something that psychotherapy would offer, which fueled my desire to work in the field and help individuals whom I felt were being ignored. In its new role as a place of treatment for the most highly symptomatic people with serious mental illnesses, Manhattan Psychiatric Center had largely surrendered its aspiration of providing state-of-the-art treatment and become a place where patients would basically sit and wait for antipsychotic medications to work.

A HATE CRIME AND THE CLOSURE OF A LIFELINE

As the 1980s shifted to the 1990s, dreams of Ward's Island serving as a place of recreation receded further into the background, as Robert Moses's footbridge was implicated in a dangerous climate that had developed on the island. In 1990 what can only be described as a hate crime rattled residents of the Keener Men's Shelter as ten to eighteen youths wearing masks walked over the footbridge on Halloween night and attacked men sleeping in the shelter with cleavers and bats, killing one man and seriously injuring nine (five people, aged thirteen to twenty-three, were later arrested for the attacks).[49] Although the crime was the most alarming and violent of its kind, it was described as following a "history of similar assaults by local youths against the homeless during the last two years."[50] An investigative article based on interviews with East Harlem and shelter residents following the crime reported that the youths detested shelter residents for their drug use, blamed them for petty crime in their neighborhood, and sought revenge. A shelter resident characterized the sentiment of local youths as bigoted, stating "they treat us like we're dogs, or dirt." The same article noted that "the attacks have left homeless men terrified, complaining that the

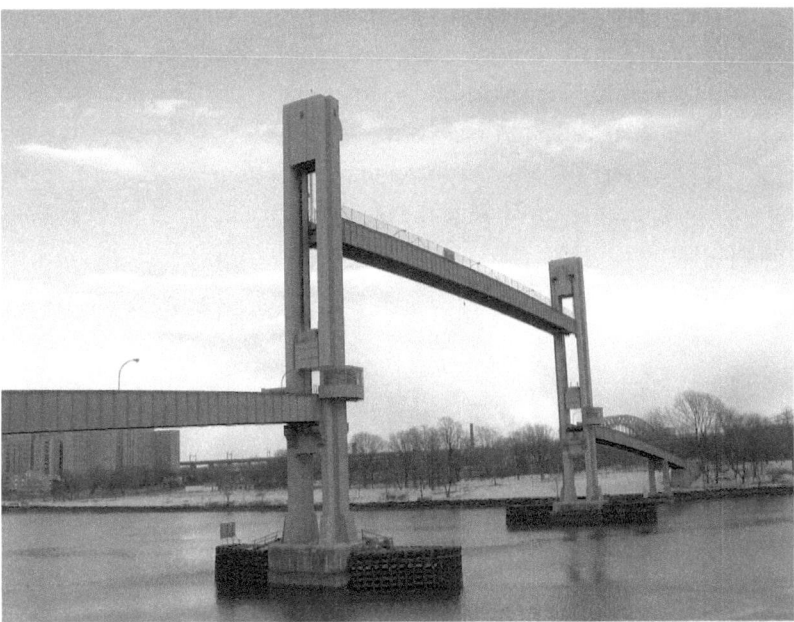

FIGURE 5.3 The Ward's Island footbridge with drawbridge raised.

Source: Wikimedia Commons.

police do not patrol the island." The evidence suggests that the attack would today meet the criteria for a hate crime, defined by the FBI as a crime "against a person or property motivated in whole or in part by an offender's bias" against a specific group. The prevalence of anti-homelessness hate crimes is discussed extensively in a 2020 report by the National Coalition for the Homeless, but there was no awareness of this type of hate crime in 1990.[51] Anti-homelessness hate crimes are described as being motivated primarily by "the perpetrator's bias against people experiencing homelessness and facilitated by their ability to target homeless people with relative ease," a description that appears to clearly fit the 1990 incident.

Although the shelter residents requested more police protection, the city's main response to the crime was instead to close the Ward's Island pedestrian bridge every night and all day from November until April, roughly half the year (see figure 5.3). The footbridge, conceived as an essential connection between East Harlem and the park, was now seen as a liability; according to a Park's Department official, "we don't get a lot of people using that bridge in the best of circumstances, and the people are not coming across it to use the parks."[52] By the early 1990s, it seemed that Ward's Island was being written off as the potential park space that Robert Moses had envisioned. But soon a dramatic turnaround would yet again change the island's place in the New York City park landscape.

6

WHERE WILL THESE CHILDREN PLAY?

By the early 1990s many in New York City had given up on restoring the city to its former grandeur. In 1992 the city recorded more than two thousand murders—a murder rate of around thirty per hundred thousand (for context, the rate in 2018 was ten times lower, at three per hundred thousand).[1] Riots occurred in 1991 and 1992 in the working- and middle-class immigrant communities of Crown Heights (in Brooklyn) and Washington Heights (in northern Manhattan), events that demoralized many inside and outside of those neighborhoods.[2] The widespread availability of crack cocaine, which peaked in the late 1980s, had ravaged several neighborhoods, both because of the direct effects of the highly addictive substance and because of the resulting acceleration of mass arrest and incarceration of people in the communities in which it was known to be distributed.[3] The HIV epidemic had hit the city hard by the early 1990s, with thousands dying every year, and the antiretroviral medications that would transform life expectancy for people who had contracted the virus were still only being researched.[4] This was the New York City of Lou Reed's popular "Dirty Blvd," a place of suffering and despair, in contrast with the romanticized picture of street life depicted in his mid-1960s song "Waiting for the Man" (mentioned in chapter 4). There was little reason to think that a place like Ward's Island, with its three psychiatric hospitals and large shelter population, would ever become the kind of urban park oasis that Robert Moses had envisioned.

Yet it was exactly at this time that a plan to remake Ward's Island began to take shape. The forces of change started in the private sector, with origins that go back to the 1980s. A 1993 article in the *New York Observer* summarized how the Manhattan private school Buckley had taken advantage of an absence of oversight and "colonized a wide swath of land on Manhattan's Wards Island, against city regulations" sometime in the early 1980s. As part of this colonization, the school maintained fields at its own expense but without permission. Buckley also employed its own private security. This led one of the school parents to decide to take on the more ambitious task of not only using and maintaining sports fields but also restoring and upgrading them. The article suggested that the City Parks Department was aware of, and turned a blind eye to, the use of public land by private schools because the parents were "deep-pocketed taxpayers."[5]

In 1992 Karen Cohen, the wife of a prominent investment banker (the former chairman of Shearson Lehman Brothers) and a parent of children from one of the schools that had been using the fields on Ward's Island, took the initiative to organize the Randall's Island Sports Foundation (RISF) as a way to formalize efforts to improve the condition of the playing fields and beautify the parkland on Ward's and neighboring Randall's Island.[6] From the beginning, the RISF was conceived as a "public-private partnership," allying the financial power of private fundraising with the political authority of the city's Parks Department. The involvement of the city's political muscle was considered essential, given the need to negotiate with the various city and state agencies that used the islands.[7] Betsy Gotbaum, the parks commissioner during the administration of Mayor David Dinkins when the RISF began, was a clear ally at the outset.[8] The alliance was further solidified when Aimee Boden, already the director of Ward's and Randall's Islands for the city's Parks Department, was appointed in a "dual capacity" as both RISF's executive director and the city's parks administrator for Ward's and Randall's Islands. Dual-capacity appointments as both directors of park foundations and employees of the Park's Department are permitted (and encouraged) based on the assumption that there is no conflict of interest between the roles.⁹

RISF set forth with an ambitious and laudable goal—to provide the children of New York City with an extensive, high-quality area in which to engage in recreation. As stated in their 2005 application for a national "urban excellence" award, "RISF was formed for the express purpose of bringing diverse agencies together to solve a problem—where will these children play."¹⁰

"INESCAPABLE" TRADEOFFS

From the outset, RISF named itself after Ward's Island's neighbor Randall's Island, even though records indicate that the use of parkland for school sports actually began on Ward's Island. RISF's effort to brand all the areas targeted for park improvement as Randall's Island and to remove the Ward's Island name whenever possible, regardless of which island they were actually on, have been clear and consistent since the organization's birth. Early documents indicate that RISF asserted that the two islands were a single entity, insisting they were "now referred to as a single 'island.'"¹¹ In RISF's current maps, unlike the official maps used by the city's Parks Department, the name Ward's is not even mentioned other than calling one area Wards Meadow Fields (see figure 6.1).¹²

It certainly makes sense that the directors of RISF would have sought to incorporate the acreage of both islands into their ambitious vision, to allow for as broad a scope as possible. However, I have been unable to locate any clear statement of the reason for their decision to focus on the Randall's Island name and act as if Ward's Island in effect no longer existed. One plausible explanation is that RISF was seeking to disassociate their focus on recreation and natural beauty from whatever institutional associations the general public had with Ward's Island. This naming pattern would be consistent with the "rebranding" of neighborhoods that is often seen in the process of urban gentrification (a

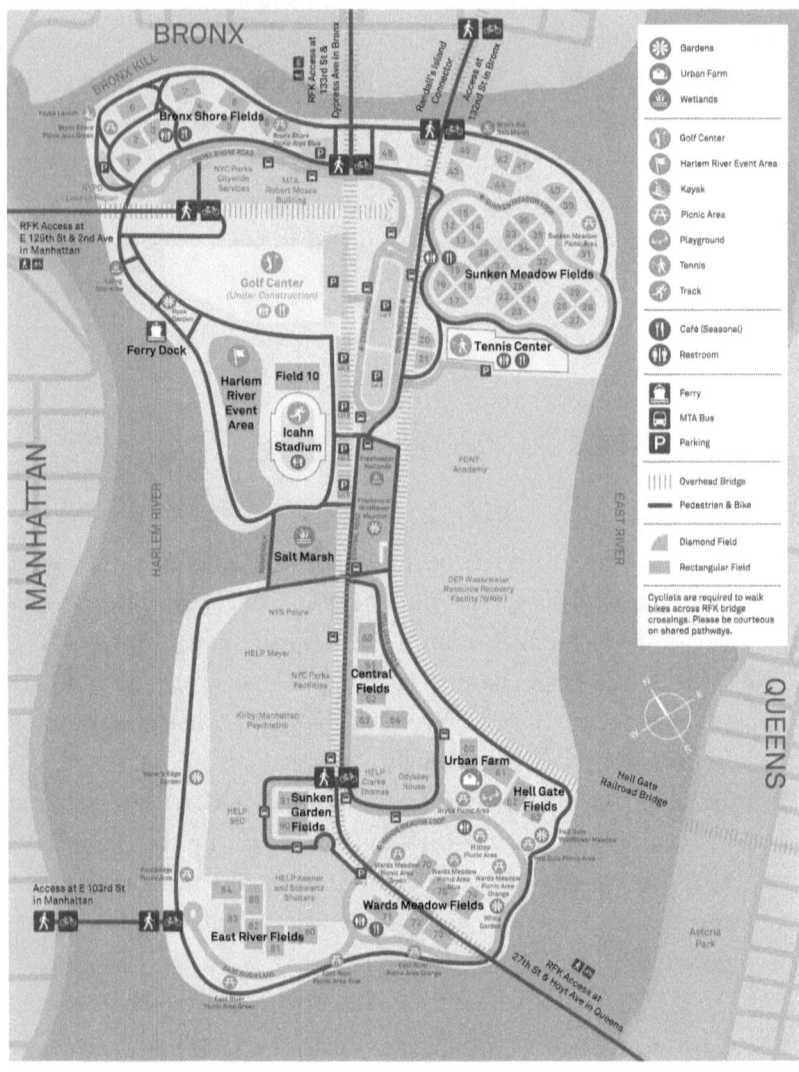

FIGURE 6.1 Map of Randall's and Ward's Islands from the Randall's Island Park Alliance website.

Source: Randall's Island Park Alliance.

national pattern that has been amply documented).[13] The logic behind rebranding can be explained by cognitive frame theory, which asserts that specific names or terms become linked with a complex set of assumptions or "scripts."[14] By disassociating an area with a name that conjures up a set of negative scripts and replacing it with a new image or "brand," real estate developers and others seek to increase the appeal of areas that might have been previously considered off-limits as places to live or visit. For example, in the Manhattan neighborhood in which I live, many property owners have sought to use the name Hudson Heights, rather than the historically rooted name of Washington Heights, because of the latter's association with drugs and crime in the 1980s and 1990s. The intentional use of the name Hudson Heights in place of the more historically rooted neighborhood name has evoked a viscerally negative reaction from many longtime residents, who see racist overtones in it.[15]

The development of Ward's Island's park resources can also be linked to the process of gentrification that was gaining steam, albeit slowly, more broadly in the 1990s.[16] The relationship between park development and gentrification has been amply documented by urban planners; it is referred to as "green gentrification."[17] A review of studies on green gentrification throughout North America has found that the development of new park spaces is strongly related to subsequent increases in property values, which can also be related to the displacement of lower-income residents. While the process by which the development of parkland leads to displacement may not be intentional, and the potentially positive impacts of parkland on the health and well-being of all residents are undeniable, green gentrification can lead to displacement, and planners need to be intentional in identifying ways to prevent it.

Concern about displacement does not appear to have been a consideration for RISF. Many early statements by its leaders indicate that they did not like the presence of institutions on Ward's Island, which they saw as a hindrance to their ambitious efforts to improve the condition of park facilities. They hoped to succeed where they believed Robert Moses had failed, eventually incorporating all of the land used by state and city institutions on Ward's Island into its ambitious park vision.[18] Karen Cohen directly stated that she hoped to claim all of Manhattan

Psychiatric Center's land for parks: "I'm a dreamer, but that's my goal... even if... we don't even have the money to do more than tear the buildings down." At best, RISF leaders saw these institutions and their residents as irrelevant to their mission to improve the park facilities on the islands. As stated in the RISF's "urban excellence" application, "certain tradeoffs are inescapable. Spatially, there must be the reallocation of certain agencies on the Island." At worst, there is evidence that the directors of RISF held disdainful attitudes toward Ward's Island's institutional residents, seeing them as human eyesores that would detract from their efforts to draw people to the newly beautified facilities. These eyesores would be best removed or at least hidden behind fences. In 1993, describing an area by the waterfront where shelter and hospital residents congregated, Aimee Boden stated "it's like 'Night of the Living Dead' back there," comparing them to zombies in the infamous 1968 horror movie.[19] She later used the same analogy in describing how the installation of fencing around Manhattan Psychiatric Center (described in chapter 1) had changed the atmosphere at the Ward's Island waterfront, repeating that "it used to be like 'Night of the Living Dead' in that corridor."[20] Statements such as these can be understood as a form of microaggressions (including assumptions of inferiority and patronization), if not more overt expressions of disdain, which I have discussed in my work on mental health stigma.[21]

Regardless of their motives, there is no question that the RISF's initiatives were successful in profoundly improving the quality of park facilities on Ward's Island. The planning for these initiatives accelerated throughout the 1990s during the administration of Mayor Rudy Giuliani, when crime began to decline rapidly (annual murders had fallen to six hundred per year by 1998) and the city's image as a crime-ridden place began to change amid the economic prosperity of the "dot-com boom."[22] During this period, plans for development were made and the city's Economic Development Corporation released "requests for expressions of interest" from contractors to complete many of the planned initiatives.[23] Goals described in a 1999 "master plan" included creating sports facilities, establishing entertainment venues, improving waterfront access, and preserving and improving parkland.

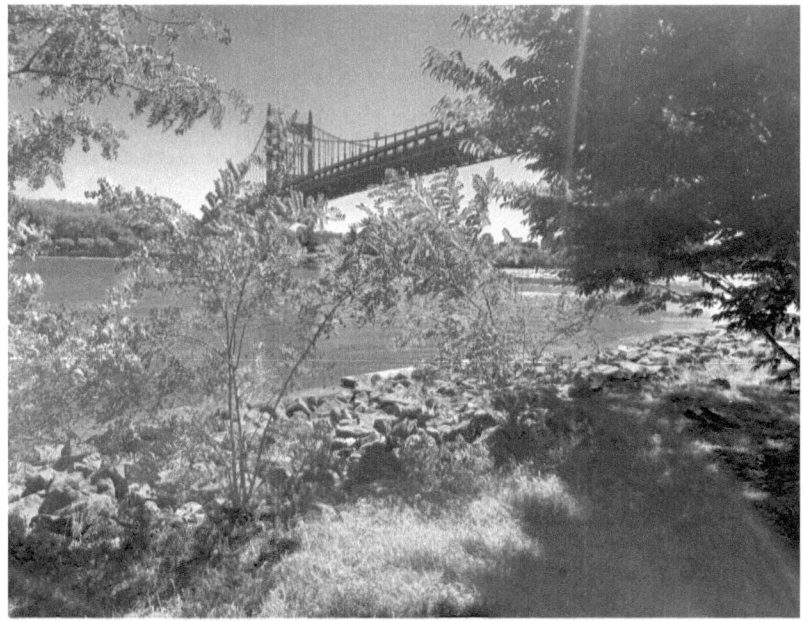

FIGURE 6.2 The Ward's Island shoreline with the Queens span of the Triborough Bridge in the distance, September 26, 2022.

Source: Photo by author.

These initiatives began to bear fruit by the early 2000s, after Michael Bloomberg became mayor, as the gentrification of many neighborhoods began to accelerate with the implementation of the Bloomberg administration's aggressive rezoning efforts.[24] The billionaire Bloomberg had been a board member of RISF before becoming mayor, and his allegiance to their mission was clearly evident after his election, as described by Karen Cohen: "having Michael Bloomberg, who was truly on our side, as mayor helped us forge ahead."[25] Although some of RISF's higher-profile initiatives (such as the replacement of Downing Stadium with more modern facilities under the name Icahn Stadium, which went on to host large concerts such as Lollapalooza and Electric Zoo, and the development of the SportTime Tennis Center) occurred on neighboring

Randall's Island, more subtle achievements included the upgrading and beautification of the sports fields, picnic areas, and shoreline on Ward's Island. A change of name, to Randall's Island Park Alliance (RIPA), in 2011 expressed this broader focus beyond sports. As indicated on their current map, facilities on Ward's Island include ten picnic areas, one playground, three gardens, and twenty-three playing fields, as well as a bike path covering the entire island shoreline (except for the area next to the Wastewater Treatment Facility).[26] Their restoration efforts produced the types of enchanting vistas seen in figure 6.2. Their efforts also led to the restoration and reopening of the footbridge (renamed the 103rd Street Footbridge on their maps, though the span itself still has a large sign that reads "Ward's Island Bridge") as a continuously available pedestrian and bicycle link between the island and East Harlem.[27] They succeeded in nearly doubling the number of visitors to the islands in the early 2000s, from 1.7 to 2.9 million visitors annually.[28]

FOR WHOSE CHILDREN? CONTROVERSY OVER PRIORITY USAGE

Although media accounts and statements from community stakeholders about RISF/RIPA's efforts were generally laudatory, their aggressive efforts were also met with controversy. As previously discussed, RISF's origin story lay in the efforts of some private schools to "lay claim" to unused fields on Ward's Island for team sports, and it is almost certain that many members of the organization's original board and donors had ties to these schools. In the early 2000s, RISF made an arrangement with a collection of private schools to provide them with "priority usage" of renovated sports fields (most on Ward's Island) from 3–6 p.m. on weekdays in exchange for a payment of $52.6 million toward the renovation. This effort received negative publicity (see figure 6.3), and a coalition of East Harlem public school parents, represented by the well-known attorney Norman Siegel, filed suit to block the initiative.[29] After the initial deal was nullified by a judge in 2008, the city and RISF/RIPA devised a new arrangement in which the private schools would be guaranteed 50 percent of the fields during after-school hours in exchange for $44 million. However, this agreement was also nullified after being reviewed by a second judge in 2009, who criticized it as an "audacious" effort to bypass the public review process.[30] As a result, the sports field renovations were paid for entirely by the Parks Department, using public funds. Parks Commissioner Adrian Benepe expressed open contempt for the decisions, saying "It was a bone-headed, ego-driven case. Our plan would have been a huge win for everyone." He also condemned what he regarded as biased media coverage and the actions of "a handful of people who had no skin in the game."[31] Regardless of the decision, by 2010 the fields were still being used primarily by private schools (56 percent of the time).

Benepe's comments notwithstanding, there is a consensus that the priority usage controversy was a blemish on the record of the RISF/RIPA,

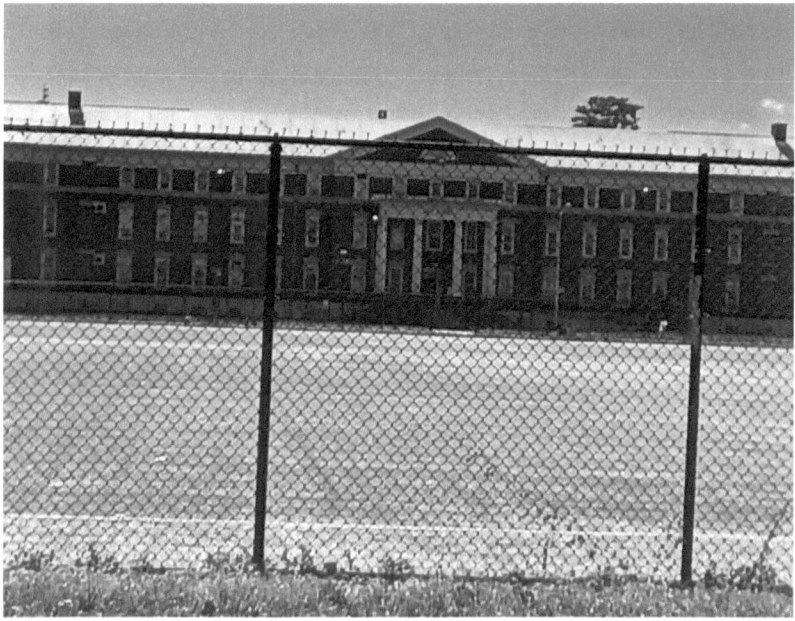

FIGURE 6.3 Renovated sports field located directly in front of the Keener Shelter, September 26, 2022.

Source: Photo by author.

as it conveyed the impression that they were not looking to benefit all the children New York City equally. Rather, they were giving priority to the children of well-off New Yorkers (the same "deep-pocketed tax payers" who founded it in 1993), whose schools could afford to support sports programs and whose parents were major donors to their initiatives and expected something in return.

BEHIND THE FENCES: INSTITUTIONAL LIFE CONTINUES AND HOMELESS SERVICES EXPAND

At the same time as RISF was fundraising and building coalitions with city agencies to expand recreational uses of Ward's Island, life went on within the institutional sectors of the island. There was some progress in reducing homelessness during the early 1990s following implementation of the collaborative city-state "New York–New York" agreement to fund housing for homeless persons with serious mental illnesses, which appears to have led to a 37 percent decrease in the city's homeless single adult homeless population (the nightly single adult average declined from 9,300 in 1989 to 6,100 in 1994).[32] However, the single adult shelter population began to increase again during the subsequent years of the Giuliani administration. Although the exact reasons for this are unclear, the Coalition for the Homeless contends this was an effect of Mayor Giuliani's decision to launch "a series of punitive policies on homeless New Yorkers," including the overpolicing of communities of color, leading to record arrest rates.[33] As a result, by the mid-1990s there was no reduction in the need to identify new locations (such as Ward's Island) in which to locate shelters, especially ones that would not generate community opposition.

In 1995 an opportunity of this kind arose when New York State governor George Pataki ordered the closure of Manhattan Children's Psychiatric Center (MCPC, opened in 1970, as we learned in chapter 4) as a budget reduction measure. At the time, MCPC housed approximately fifty children and also served a hundred children in its outpatient program.³⁴ Concurrently, the city was proposing to locate a new shelter in a large armory space in the middle-class neighborhood of Flushing, Queens, but community members and local elected officials opposed the plan and suggested that the soon-to-be-vacant buildings of MCPC be used instead.³⁵ The lack of a local "community" on the island was seen to be a strength of the location, as reflected in a statement attributed to an elected official's aide: "the psychiatric center, on the west side of Ward's Island, could be a better site because it is not surrounded by businesses and residential neighborhoods." Within a few months, documents from the Giuliani administration indicated that they had moved forward into negotiating with New York State for the use of the Manhattan Children's Psychiatric Center buildings to create a new "250 beds" in collaboration with the nonprofit organization HELP USA.³⁶ In these documents, it was noted that using this site would "resolve community concerns." The resulting shelter opened within a year; later called the Clarke Thomas Men's Shelter, it housed two hundred men (see figure 6.4). The opening of this shelter brought the overall shelter population on Ward's Island close to nine hundred by the end of the 1990s.

Interestingly, although concurrent documents from the Giuliani administration discussed Ward's and Randall's Island being "referred

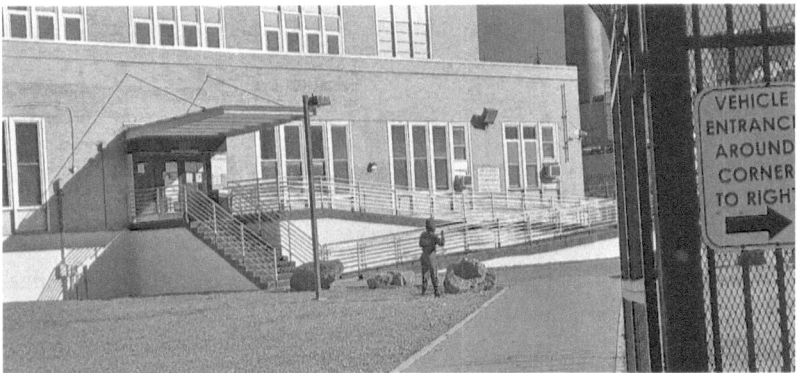

FIGURE 6.4 Clarke Thomas Men's Shelter, November 20, 2023.

Source: Photo by author.

to as a single 'island,'" documents about the opening of the prospective shelter referred to its location categorically as "Ward's Island."[37] It seems that the Ward's Island name would continue to be used whenever referring to the institutional locations on the island.

RENOVATION AT ODYSSEY HOUSE

In chapter 4 we saw that Odyssey House had started a program for mothers and children in a former hospital building in the early 1970s (the Mabon building). Records indicate that they continued to serve two hundred people at the site: a sixty-bed facility for mothers and children, in addition to a 140-bed residential substance use treatment program for young adults. Sometime in the 1990s, it was determined that the Mabon building, originally built in 1915, was in desperate need of renovation, but it appears to have continued to operate throughout the 1990s and 2000s. An article from 2002 discussed how a survivor of the 9/11 attacks was able to receive support at Odyssey House's Ward's Island facility.[38] The Mabon building eventually received a substantial renovation and upgrade in the 2010s with support from the New York State Office of Addiction Supports and Services (OASAS).[39]

PSYCHIATRIC REHABILITATION ARRIVES AT MANHATTAN PSYCHIATRIC CENTER

Meanwhile, at Manhattan Psychiatric Center, the census continued to decline, with state records indicating that the hospital's census had declined to 883 in 1992 and roughly 700 in 1999.[40] Amid this census decline, the core group of people served by the state hospital became increasingly characterized by special needs that complicated treatment, including substance use co-occurrence, homelessness, and forensic (criminal justice) involvement. Records from the early 1990s indicate that roughly 30 percent of that inpatient population had one of these special needs. These clients were predominantly men and people of color (Black and Latino/a/x). At the same time, there is evidence that the innovations of the psychiatric rehabilitation movement and an increasing focus on what was now being termed mental health recovery had finally begun to arrive at the state hospital system.[41] This recovery vision saw the mission of the public mental health services system as helping people to manage the symptoms of mental illness with the goal of living lives of their own choosing in the community.[42] Although this vision was similar to the optimistic vision evident in reports from the 1950s and early 1960s, it was accompanied by a more concrete evidence base for the types of services that could facilitate recovery. Psychiatric rehabilitation services, which embraced recovery, focused on teaching people specific skills needed to cope with symptoms and stress in order to facilitate community living.

Records indicate that Manhattan Psychiatric Center began implementing psychiatric rehabilitation services, with a particular focus on addressing the needs of people who had experienced criminal justice involvement, sometime in the 1990s. In 1997 the hospital initiated the STAIR (Service for Treatment and Abatement of Interpersonal Risk) program, a cognitive skills training program focused on addressing the needs of patients with a history of prior incarceration. In contrast to the lack of structure and aimlessness described in the 1980s New York State Commission on Quality of Care for the Mentally Disabled report (described in chapter 5), STAIR was highly structured and organized. The program consisted of seventy-two small group sessions delivered over the course of six months. Groups sessions were run by trained clinicians and taught cognitive techniques including "problem solving, creative thinking, values enhancement, improvement of social skills, use of critical reasoning, and managing emotions." The report on the first 181 persons engaged in the program indicated that the program was reaching predominantly African American men with histories of substance use and multiple arrests.[43]

Although it is not known if he participated in the STAIR program, a famous resident of Manhattan Psychiatric Center during this period was

Russell Jones, better known as Ol' Dirty Bastard, a member of the legendary Staten Island hip-hop collective Wu Tang Clan.[44] A friend reported that "nobody helped him, nobody visited him" while he was hospitalized.[45] Jones spoke very little about the experience but is reported to have referred to it as a "hellhole hotel." Jones died in 2004 of an accidental drug overdose.

By the early 2010s Ward's Island had arrived at a place of dual identity. It was now home to a legion of sports fields, bike paths, and picnic grounds that had finally reached a point of widespread use among general community members (many of them students at expensive private schools, primarily from affluent backgrounds) and, at the same time, served almost two thousand of society's most marginalized people—the majority of them people of color with serious mental illness and a history of substance use, homelessness or housing instability, and incarceration—in a range of institutional settings. Park spaces and institutional settings were separated by high fences, providing a physical and psychological barrier between the two worlds. An uneasy détente had been arrived at—but was it sustainable?

7

"WE ARE NEW YORK'S FORGOTTEN PEOPLE"

The Island Now

By the 2010s there was a dramatic change in Ward's Island's image, driven by the initiatives led by the Randall's Island Sports Foundation/Park Alliance (RISF/RIPA). These efforts were successful in finally bringing large numbers of New Yorkers to the island for recreation, as Robert Moses had envisioned in the 1930s but was unable to achieve during his lifetime. They have been so successful, in fact, that many New Yorkers have the impression that Ward's Island no longer exists, that it is instead just an extension of its more consistently park-oriented neighbor, Randall's Island. This is reflected in maps of the island (shown in chapter 6) that show the areas where people live in institutions in the same manner as the Wastewater Treatment Facility—as a no-go gray zone.

At the same time, despite the best efforts of RISF/RIPA, there has been very little decline in the number of people residing in the island's institutional facilities. As established by the late 1990s, at the time of this writing (late 2023) the island is currently the location of seven institutions:

- Two large shelters focused on men with mental health conditions (Clarke Thomas and Keener), housing 500 people in total (a third

shelter, the 200-bed HELP USA men's shelter, located within one of the buildings of Manhattan Psychiatric Center, opened in 2019 but quickly shuttered in 2022 because of structural problems).[1]
- Two state psychiatric hospitals (Manhattan Psychiatric Center and Kirby Forensic Psychiatric Center), currently housing roughly 350 people in total.
- The Odyssey House residential substance use facility (renovated in 2017 and now called the George Rosenfeld Center for Recovery) housing roughly 250 people.[2]
- Manhattan Psychiatric Center's Transitional Living Residence and a community residence for people diagnosed with mental illnesses managed by the Jewish Board for Family and Children's Services, housing roughly 120 people in total

In the 2010 census, the island's total population was listed as 1,648, with 100 percent of the island's residents living in "group quarters," a percentage that is singular among New York City census tracts. Consistent with what we have seen in previous chapters, the great majority were Black and Latino/a/x (52 percent and 33 percent, respectively). In the 2020 census, its total population declined somewhat to 1,302, but this seems to have been solely the result of a decline in the census of the two hospitals. As in 2010, all of the island's residents lived in group-based settings, although a small number (eighty-six in total) were identified as living in "households" (presumably families residing together in the reopened Odyssey House facility). The island's residents remained predominantly Black and Latino/a/x (48 percent and 36 percent, respectively).[3]

Ward's Island can thus be characterized as having a dual identity. One component of this identity is referred to as Randall's Island and features renovated parkland that serves predominantly privileged children and families, many affiliated with the private schools that are the primary users of its sports fields, as described in the last chapter. The image here is of wide-open space, beautiful views, and high-quality sports facilities. The other identity, which continues to be called Ward's Island (in official documents, as the announced route of the M35 bus, by residents, and by those who work at service sites), features drab and decaying buildings.[4] The image here is of an urban exile, with poor living conditions, no services, and infrequent public transportation. The buildings serve as a place of residence for society's most dispossessed: predominantly people of color, currently or recently homeless, almost all with psychiatric histories, many with substance use histories, and many with histories of criminal justice involvement. An important consideration in current studies of stigma is "intersectionality," and it is hard to imagine a group that embodies more intersecting stigmatized categories than these individuals.[5] An overhead view of the island neatly encapsulates this dual identity (see figure 7.1).

Although I have not seen the term "dual identity" used with reference to other cities, several researchers have referred to the issue of "contested spaces" in gentrifying cities.[6] These contested spaces are often areas, such as parks and squares, that have been historically used by a lower-income groups who are then pressured to leave them, through implicit and explicit means, to "cater to the needs and interests of middle class and elite users." This process was first described in Chicago by sociologist

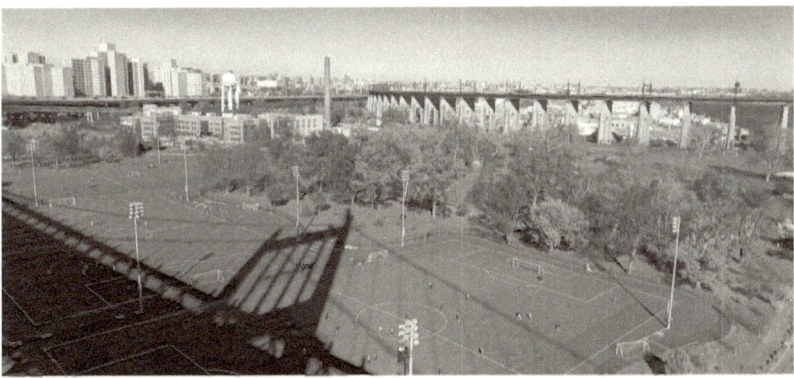

FIGURE 7.1 View of Ward's Island from the Robert F. Kennedy Bridge pedestrian path, November 20, 2023. Note the large open playing fields and the brick buildings crowded together beyond.

Source: Photo by author.

Talmadge Wright, and has since been documented as playing out in cities throughout North America and Europe.[7] Lower-income groups may experience exclusion in contested spaces as they come to feel that they are being driven out of the city. The perspectives of both higher- and lower-income residents are of interest in trying to understand contested spaces, and I sought to understand the views of both in my exploration of how Ward's Island is currently seen.

AWARENESS OF THE ISLAND BY NEW YORK CITY RESIDENTS

Although it might be expected, given the island's popularity as a place of sports and recreation, that most New Yorker would be aware of Ward's Island's residents, evidence suggests that most are completely unaware of their existence. In an online survey of 284 New York City residents that I conducted in late 2022, roughly 63 percent reported that they had either "never heard" of Ward's Island or were "unsure" if they had.[8] When asked to write in what they thought was located on the island, the most typical response (given by 36 percent of respondents) was "no response." Only 7 percent of respondents overall were able to correctly identify the island as the location of both hospitals and shelters, while 31 percent gave a response that was judged as "partially correct." Many of these partially correct responses indicated that respondents were aware only of the park facilities on the island: "I know it's mostly used for park activities and outside festivals." Many partially correct responses showed an awareness that the island had a *history* of institutions but a belief that these were a thing of the past.[9] Illustrative responses included:

"There used to be a psychiatric facility."

"Is this the island that once held a hospital for smallpox, but has been mostly abandoned?"

"It sounds like one of those islands that used to be a hospital."

"I think there are old buildings that are no longer in use. Maybe an old military base or hospital."

"Sounds like it has a prison facility on it. I am unsure if people live there."

Thus, many New Yorkers have a vague sense that the island has a historical institutional connection but are unaware of any direct association with the present day, let alone that it still houses multiple institutions serving more than a thousand people. (Other responses were flatly incorrect but conveyed the sense that the island had some kind of institutional history: "I think it was the island used as quarantine for a disease and was host to 'Typhoon Mary.'")

In the same survey, I asked participants if they had heard of Randall's Island, and 67 percent responded affirmatively. Respondents were clear that Randall's Island was a place of recreation, with illustrative responses including "there's soccer fields and a bridge over it. I don't think its residential"; and "sports facilities, like baseball/softball fields." The clear discrepancy between awareness of Ward's and Randall's Islands indicates that RISF/RIPA has been largely successful in making the public much more aware of Randall's Island and making parkland and sports facilities the primary association in the public's consciousness.

ATTENTION TO SHELTER RESIDENTS DURING COVID-19

As will be familiar to most readers, New York City was one of the epicenters of the COVID-19 pandemic during its early phase in 2020, with city residents who were "older, had underlying medical conditions, or resided in poorer neighborhoods, and racial and ethnic minority populations" suffering "disproportionately from [COVID-19] infection and death."[10] This was partly related to the fact that many of these poorer residents continued to work in "essential" in-person service occupations or lived in more crowded quarters with others who worked in these occupations, while more affluent city residents were able to work remotely and/or had fled to suburban or rural areas away from the epicenter.[11] Among the high-risk groups, people living in congregate settings with minimal space separation, such as shelters, were at even greater risk of infection, and people with serious mental illnesses were subsequently found to be at significantly greater risk of death when infected (the reasons are unclear but may be related to elevated rates of somatic comorbidities in this group).[12]

Given awareness of the multiple COVID-19 risk factors borne by shelter residents, especially those with serious mental illness, there was some attention paid to the conditions of Ward's Island's shelters during the height of the COVID-19 pandemic. An article published in 2020 in the online magazine *The City* reported on the strained atmosphere within crowded shelters, including those on Ward's Island.[13] An article published in mid-2021 in the free newspaper *The Villager/AM New York* provided a more detailed report on a visit by New York City public advocate Jumaane Williams and other elected officials to shelters on the island (note that the location of the shelters was clearly identified as "Ward's Island").[14] The article included testimonials from shelter residents decrying the absence of services on the island, the infrequency of the M35 bus, and substandard conditions within the shelters themselves. One Clarke Thomas shelter resident stated: "People should never live like this! It's wrong." A formerly homeless advocate joining the visit eloquently stated that the fact that they were living in housing of last resort "does not give you the right to dehumanize us . . . that does not give you the right to put us here and warehouse us for years, where we lose our sense of self, we lose our sense of wanting to go out and be productive members of society." A related report published in another online outlet about the same visit highlighted the isolation of the island: "You have to get on a bus into Manhattan to do anything. . . . You're away from everybody.... When they put you here, it's usually to forget about you."[15] Photos were shared of the poor living conditions within the shelter; they revealed clearly how little privacy residents have, as well their small beds and the dilapidated condition of the building. Although these quotes and photos speak to fundamental aspects of life on Ward's Island that existed long before (and continue to persist after) the COVID-19 crisis, the elected officials visiting seemed most concerned with pandemic-related issues. The article noted that Public Advocate Williams "found the lack of on-site services and COVID-19 protections to be the most troubling." Thus, the fundamental reality of life on Ward's Island—that it is in a remote location with a complete absence of services—was not challenged, even by the politically progressive Williams. It should also be noted that these articles were published in relatively obscure outlets; with the exception of an article in the conservative tabloid the *New York Post*, the visit was not reported on by more mainstream media outlets.[16]

THE EXPERIENCE OF LIVING ON THE ISLAND

The above referenced media reports present an emphatically negative impression of what life on Ward's Island is like, but they of course might be biased by the agenda of the journalists authoring the accounts. I therefore decided to collect original data to inform an understanding of the experience of people living on the island. In the spring of 2023, I received approval to conduct brief qualitative interviews with randomly approached current residents about their experiences.[17] Recruitment was conducted by outdoor outreach with residents as they were waiting to take the M35 bus or hanging around in public areas. Residents interviewed provided informed consent and were compensated for their participation with twenty-dollar gift cards.[18] In addition to questions probing opinions about the availability of amenities and public transportation on the island, participants were asked open-ended questions intended to help us understand their experience, including: "Please describe, in your own words, what it's like for you to live/stay on Ward's Island" and "What would you like New Yorkers who are unfamiliar with it to know about Ward's Island and what it's like to live on it?"

We surveyed a total of twenty-eight island residents, split roughly evenly between persons living in one of the shelters or one of the community housing facilities (either the Transitional Living Residence or the Jewish Board residence). Demographically, they were similar to the people experiencing homelessness in New York City: middle-aged (a mean age of forty-eight), predominantly male (92 percent), and predominantly people of color (61 percent Black, 21 percent Latino/a). Participants had resided on the island for varying lengths of time, from one month to ten years (with a mean of roughly 2.5 years). Interview responses were coded by two independent raters and organized into themes after a consensus review of their categories. The most commonly endorsed themes were negative, including lack of resources (mentioned in fifteen responses), dangerous conditions (eleven responses), unsanitary conditions (seven responses), and awareness of separation between residents and nonresidents (four responses). As to what they would like New Yorkers to know about Ward's Island, one participant provided a clear and powerful response consistent with the media reports: "The Goddamn truth. We are New York's forgotten people, discarded, not treated like people." This response communicates an awareness that living in a remote location was a consequence of wanting to "keep people away," a major driver of stigma, as discussed in chapter 1.[19]

Regarding the extent to which they perceived they might have access to some of the amenities created by RISF/RIPA, one participant clearly stated the understanding that they were not welcome: "We don't go over there because of our label, not because we'll start a fight. It's protected. This place is separate from the bicycle place." The high fences erected to prevent the bike path from looking like "Night of the Living Dead" not only served as a physical barrier but also conveyed a clear psychological message: "stay away"; "you are not welcome"; "this is for other, more worthy, people." Again, this communicates an awareness of being a member of a stigmatized community being kept away from more "deserving" members of society.

Finally, a response representative of the type categorized as "lack of resources" was "You have to wait for the bus just to go to the store."

Alongside these predominantly negative responses, however, some positive themes that did not appear in any of the media accounts were endorsed, sometimes within the same interviews. These included "enjoys park space" (mentioned in seven responses) and "Ward's Island offers comfort and peace" (three responses). Some illustrative quotes are "Ward's Island is a special place" and "This island is a good space for your mind."

These responses suggest that many residents do appreciate the natural beauty and sense of sanctuary that residence on Ward's Island provides and that this aspect of life there should not be ignored. They also resonate with my experience of living on the island as a child, finding it to be a place of "comfort and peace" on many occasions.

THE EXPERIENCE OF WORKING ON THE ISLAND

I also received approval to conduct interviews with individuals who had recently worked as treatment staff at Manhattan Psychiatric Center or Kirby Forensic Psychiatric Center to obtain their perspectives on what it was like to work on Ward's Island. Six former staff members, ranging in age from thirty-seven to seventy-five, whose job roles included recreational therapist, direct care counselor, psychology trainee, and psychologists participated in these qualitative interviews.[20]

One former psychologist described the experience of working on the island as "intense": "It was always a kind of an intense experience. You know, when you're on the island, it sort of felt very different from being in another part of the city and being a part of these big institutions, behind double razor wire fences and all the fences. I mean, it was sort of a community of people there. It seemed kind of separated and isolated from the rest of Manhattan."

A former recreational art therapist voiced a sense of isolation: "It's very isolated out there. There's almost nowhere to get anything except for at the actual hospital."

A former psychology trainee described being aware of the profound disconnect between residents of the island and the community members who use it for recreation. They described the contrast between the revelry of attendees at a music festival and the drab institutional life of island residents in a manner similar to what I described in chapter 1: "There was a huge music festival, a rave. So you have all these 20 something year olds coming to the Island getting ready to party literally right next door to Manhattan Psychiatric Center. And so they heard everything and it was just such a dichotomy. Here are these people who probably spent so much money to buy these tickets and then I don't even think they knew what was happening next door. They just saw this big beige building. So that was definitely a very stark and vivid memory I have of my time there."

These responses suggest that staff, like residents, are aware of the disconnect between the way that New York's more privileged residents experience the island and the experience of those who live there.

CURRENT CONDITIONS WITHIN MANHATTAN PSYCHIATRIC CENTER

Since its early days, Manhattan Psychiatric Center (the direct descendent of the New York City Asylum for the Insane) has been Ward's Island's most consistent tenant. As we saw in chapter 2, the asylum/hospital started out with a census of roughly five hundred in 1875 and grew rapidly until reaching more than eight thousand in 1930. The numbers have declined steadily since then, first because of forced transfers related to the expectation that the hospital would be compelled to close in the 1940s and then because of deinstitutionalization. At the time of this writing, the census of Manhattan Psychiatric Center has reached a near all-time low average daily census of 152. Patients who are admitted (like

Carlos, whom I spoke about in chapter 1) tend to stay for lengthy periods. The median length of stay for those discharged within a year is three hundred days (approximately ten months); nearly half of patients are categorized as "long stay," or more than one year.[21] Neighboring Kirby Forensic Psychiatric Center has a slightly higher census of 206 but a shorter median length of stay. For those discharged within a year, it is 155 days (approximately five months), but half of patients there are also categorized as "long stay." Thus, at any point in time, there are roughly 350 persons housed in the two inpatient facilities on the island.

The service mission of the hospitals today is a far cry from the original asylum's general mission of serving the city's "indigent insane." For context, the hospitals serve only .1 percent of the roughly 325,000 people receiving public-sector services from facilities licensed by the New York State Office of Mental Health in New York City.[22] By their own description, the hospitals serve a high-need population with "multiple disadvantages in the form of social and educational deprivation, physical disabilities, intellectual/cognitive impairment, trauma histories, substance misuse, and legal system involvement."[23] Manhattan Psychiatric Center reports that the patient population remains primarily persons of color, with nearly half (49 percent) identifying as Black, 19 percent as white, 8 percent as Hispanic/Latino/a/x, and 9 percent as Asian. The services at the inpatient facilities, which were historically underresourced, are now generously funded, with the cost of housing an inpatient conservatively estimate at $1,136 per day (more than $400,000 per year), based on state-reported "standard charges" for inpatient services.[24]

What types of services are offered at the hospitals? Based on its own description, Manhattan Psychiatric Center now requires all patients to participate in groups at the "treatment malls," an area separate from the units where they eat and sleep. They explicitly describe the atmosphere as "school-like and progress oriented," in contrast to the "often custodial-type programs given on the home wards in the past."[25] Groups offered in the treatment malls focus on the evidence-based Wellness Self-Management program, which "follows a manualized psychoeducational program utilizing multiple teaching modules, including education about the disease, the medication, health and wellness."[26] Most or all patients also participate in another evidence-based intervention, cognitive remediation.[27] Designed to help improve specific areas of cognition, such as memory, attention, and processing speed, that are frequently affected among people with serious mental illnesses, this program includes targeted computerized tasks aimed at improving these cognitive skills. Dr. J. P. Lindenmayer, one of the hospital's psychiatrists, has coauthored several peer-reviewed articles documenting the effectiveness of cognitive remediation administered to patients recruited through the hospital.[28] The manual for the hospital's psychology internship program also describes the use of individual cognitive behavioral therapy,[29] another evidence-based practice, with inpatients within specialized Transition to Home units housing individuals who were recently homeless,[30] as well as dialectical behavior therapy (DBT) in groups.[31] All of these approaches are consistent with current standards for evidence-based treatment of severe mental illness.

As previously noted, my research team conducted interviews with former hospital staff to understand their perspective on the service environment at the island's hospitals. I also asked them about their impressions of the quality of services offered at Manhattan Psychiatric Center and Kirby and whether they believed that the services offered were evidence-based and/or cutting-edge. The former staff members we interviewed generally agreed that the hospital was providing good-quality services.

A former psychology trainee at the hospital stated: "I would say they actually did a decent job offering things like cognitive remediation, some DBT skills training groups.... There was an evidence-based trauma-informed approach that the staff were trained in. So wouldn't say it was cutting edge, but I would say it was definitely in line with professional standards and recommendations for this population."

Another former psychologist described the services in a manner very similar to how they were described by the hospital's self-characterization: "They provide psychopharmacology, they provide individual group therapy, they provide rehab therapy, and the goal is to help people to a point in recovery where they can leave the hospital and go back to living in the community, and the services there were great. I think that, it's a state hospital, so there might have been some issues with resources and funding, but people were definitely great and the staff was great and they really tried to make the best out of what they had."

Another former staff person at Kirby Forensic agreed: "I wouldn't say it was cutting-edge, I think it was evidence-based. We did the CBT type of groups."

A participant who had worked at Manhattan Psychiatric Center starting in the 1980s indicated that the hospital had shown a significant evolution in its perspective toward its role over that time span, stating:

> I felt that the ancillary services, the treatment mall, and the groups that they were decided to participate in, were excellent preparations for being back in the community. . . . I felt that it was enormously valuable and it was one of the biggest improvements that MPC provided from the time that I came, which was essentially, these are patients who have not been able to succeed in the community, because of the severity of their symptomatology. . . . The first ward I was on, [a staff member] prided herself in not discharging patients because she came from the viewpoint that these were people who needed to be institutionalized, who would benefit most greatly from our providing the sanctuary of being away from the stresses of the community.

These responses affirm that, though their role has evolved to serve only a small and very high need segment of people with severe mental illnesses (many with histories of criminal justice involvement), the state hospitals located on Ward's Island have arrived at a place where they are now providing high-quality, evidence-based services that might be considered worthy of what Dr. Koz envisioned in the 1970s—"they should get the best care, not the worst."

THE INTRODUCTION OF A SHELTER FOR ASYLUM SEEKERS

In addition to the institutions previously described, at the time of this writing (in late 2023 and early 2024), a new element—but one that harks back to the island's origin story as an "emigrant refuge"—has been introduced into the mix on Ward's Island: a two-thousand-bed tent-based temporary shelter for international asylum seekers. (As this book goes to press, it is reported that the shelter will be closed in early 2025).[32] It was opened in August 2023 amid a rapid influx of asylum seekers coming to New York City (either of their own accord or bused by the governors of southern border states). Large numbers of the asylum seekers have come from Venezuela after making the long trek through Central America and Mexico, but many others have traveled from West Africa and China.[33] The shelter consists of a large series of tents erected atop four soccer fields located behind the Keener Men's Shelter.[34] With tents looming so large that they are visible from across the East River, this shelter has more than doubled the island's population overnight (see figure 7.2). Even though it is clearly located on Ward's Island, city leaders inexplicably and consistently have chosen to refer to the location as Randall's Island, and media outlets have not questioned this.

There was a modest amount of opposition to the announcement of the opening of the shelter. However, compared to other areas of the city, where the decision to site migrant shelters was met to with open and vitriolic protests, these responses were only minimally negative or even favorable.[35] One parent quoted in the *New York Times* spoke of the loss

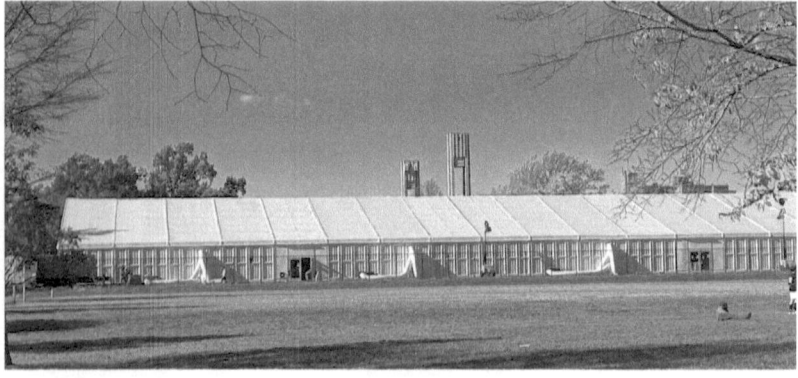

FIGURE 7.2 Migrant tent shelter on Ward's Island, November 20, 2023.

Source: Photo by author.

of soccer fields as an inconvenience that was overridden by the urgent need for housing: "If that means that some people miss a few practices for some period of time . . . I think that's a perfectly reasonable thing to give, if it means that a lot of people have somewhere to sleep."[36] This response is in stark contrast to a statement from a protester against the opening of a shelter in Brooklyn, suggesting that the shelter was a threat to public safety: "This is our battle for our neighborhoods, for our children, for our grandparents." One factor in these differing responses is the general political preference of the voters in the areas near Ward's Island (predominantly liberal Democrat), in contrast with more conservative Democrats and Republicans is some of the areas of Brooklyn and Queens where protests have taken place, but another is the simple fact that, going back to the late 1840s, opening large institutions on Ward's Island has not produced significant community opposition because the island does not have a "community" that can rise up in opposition.

That is to say, with the exception of the existing shelter residents. When preparations were made to open a migrant shelter on Randall's Island proper in late 2022, a local news channel reported that two residents of the Clarke Thomas Men's Shelter took exception to what they perceived as the preferential treatment afforded residents of the migrant shelter. The men were quoted as saying, "We get treated bad. They get treated better than us," noting that men at the migrant center were provided with a "recreation room with multiple TVs, plush couches, telephones for calling home, Xbox, foosball tables and games," while the recreation room at Clarke Thomas has "a single TV and uncomfortable, molded plastic chairs."[37] Other media outlets also carried this story, largely with an emphasis on why the migrants were being treated so well rather than why the Clarke Thomas residents were being treated so poorly.

Reporting on the opposition of the "home-grown" homeless to recent asylum seekers might simply reflect an opportunistic attempt by media outlets to stir outrage about preferential treatment being given to "non-Americans." However, there is also plausibly an element of truth to the suggestion of preferential treatment if city authorities see the migrants as a "more deserving" category than the frequently justice-involved and

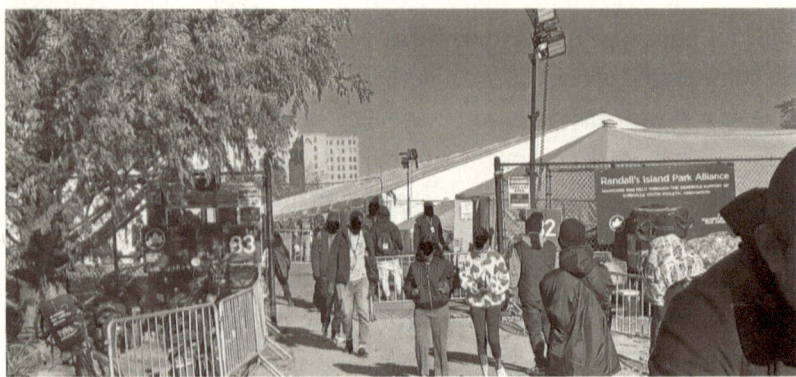

FIGURE 7.3 Entrance to the migrant tent shelter on Ward's Island, November 20, 2023.

Source: Photo by author.

substance-using persons who live on Ward's Island.[38] Otherwise, why state that the shelter would be located on the less stigmatized Randall's Island than on Ward's Island, where it actually was?

My recent journey to Ward's Island suggested to me that there are, in fact, two worlds of shelter residents on Ward's Island. On a sunny fall day, in front of the Keener and Clarke Thomas shelters, few people could be seen congregating outside enjoying the island's beauty, with residents presumably either inside or having taken the M35 bus to Harlem. Outside the migrant shelter, however, the area teemed with life (see figure 7.3). Consistent with what has been reported in the media, impromptu businesses appeared to have sprung up, selling coffee, food, and other goods that are unavailable on the island.[39] Residents of the migrant shelter could be seen coming and going and sitting outside enjoying the sunshine. As I walked over the footbridge to Manhattan, I was passed by many apparent migrant shelter residents on electric bikes and scooters, likely traveling to delivery jobs. Life in the migrant shelter is clearly a challenge (as can be imagined and as is described in media accounts), but this was still a different feeling than I have previously had on the island—it felt something like a community.

My experience and the reports of how existing shelter residents perceive being treated differently raise the question of whether it is possible for the island to be host to a more formal community of this kind. I will address this question in the next chapter, which will consider the possible future of Ward's Island.

8

THE FUTURE

What Can Ward's Island Become?

As we have seen throughout this book, from the time it was acquired by New York City in the 1840s to the present day, Ward's Island has never been part of the mainstream of New York society. It now sits as a "contested space" uncomfortably at the juncture of two identities, serving two distinct and unrelated purposes: on the one hand, as a place of daytime recreation for various groups (mostly school-based) and, on the other, as a place of residence for more than a thousand of society's most marginalized people. It has managed to maintain the second part of its identity despite concerted efforts by a number of powerful figures and interest groups to evict its institutions for the past hundred years. A crosscutting theme throughout the island's history is that it has primarily served as a home for society's most disadvantaged, those experiencing systemic oppression and social exclusion. Beginning in the 1800s, the island's residents were predominantly recent immigrants; the residents of Manhattan State Hospital were consistently reported to be "foreign born." Today the residents of the island's hospitals and shelters are primarily Black and Latino men, groups that have been disproportionately targeted by America's unequal justice system. It is also currently home to a large number of recent asylum seekers from South America and West Africa. Both of these groups have encountered, and continue to arouse, intense community opposition when provided with housing in other parts of the city. The city's need for a location where marginalized people can be quickly placed without concern for community opposition remains a powerful force driving the island's ongoing use as a place of urban exile.

What of the future? Will Ward's Island remain in this dual role indefinitely, will one of its identities come to predominate, or is there another way for this unique location to benefit the people of New York City? In this chapter, I discuss two competing visions and then explore a possibly alternate vision for the island's future that centers the interests of the people who currently live (and have always lived) there—low-income people diagnosed with serious mental illnesses.

ONE VISION

As I discussed in chapter 6, RISF/RIPA has made clear its intention to achieve Robert Moses's vision of removing all institutions from Ward's Island and converting the reclaimed space to parkland. This vision was articulated in official materials distributed to New York City government in the 1990s, which listed as a goal the "eventual removal/relocation of disruptive, inappropriate park land uses" including "homeless shelters" and "Odyssey House."[1] The goal of closing Manhattan Psychiatric Center was also expressed clearly in the 2011 edition of *The Other Islands of New York City*, which quoted the RISF/RIPA founder Karen Cohen as stating that it was her goal to close or move the hospital "even if in my lifetime we don't even have the money to do more than tear the buildings down."[2]

Would those who provide services to the high-need individuals currently served on Ward's Island be in favor of relocating them? I decided to explore how stakeholders in the mental health community would feel about the possibility of relocating services from Ward's Island to other areas and the conversion of these areas to parkland. As will be recalled from chapter 7, members of my research team conducted qualitative interviews with six former staff members whose job roles included recreational therapist, direct care counselor, psychology trainee, and psychologist. When asked what they thought about the closure of current service facilities on the island and their conversion to parkland, they gave emphatically negative responses.[3]

One former direct care counselor responded with outrage, stating: "No, they can't do that. They can't do that. No, they can't do that. Them people need those places. You see how the homeless, the epidemic of the homelessness, and psychiatric carries out here in the city? Oh, they can't do that. They need to keep them places and they need to help these people more. Nobody, like they don't do no outreach. They need to come out and see how these people are living."

Similarly, a former psychologist stated: "I think that's a terrible idea. I think there are already outcasts and they have very little place to be and that's a very small refuge for them to be in, and it's very much needed and that would be a terrible loss of services."

Another former psychologist opined that the motivation for such an initiative would be the same one that had led to locating the institutions on Ward's Island in the first place ("keeping people away"), taken a step further: "People in society tend to not want to deal with the mentally ill, they are one of the most stigmatized population, and just that they want to say that, why can't they integrate the population of Manhattan's Psychiatric Center into that? Is that that they won't—I think that that's horrible and I think that it discounts the humanity of the people on that Island. So I think it's a terrible idea."

Finally, another former psychologist linked its motivation to the selfish economic motives considered in chapter 6: "It sounds like taking what could be a potentially nice environment, making it better, and kicking out the people who could really benefit from it. I would love to have the people that have the same services, but have them more integrated into having it be a park-like setting. Again, they could be living there and mowing the lawn, and learning horticulture, and being things like that. I think that would be not a good—just another gentrification, really?"

Though finding Ward's Island to be remote and lacking services, these stakeholders still see it as fulfilling an important role in New York

City's service landscape, and the idea of relocating services to other areas elicits a viscerally negative response. This negative response likely also stems from prior experiences of broken promises and the expectation that, when something is taken away, it is not actually replaced.

Removing institutions from Ward's Island would not necessarily mean that the needs of its residents would be abandoned. It could certainly be argued that it would be in their interest to have their psychiatric and shelter-based needs addressed in other parts of the city that are more accessible to resources that are nonexistent on the island. Further, the hypothetical closure of Manhattan Psychiatric Center would free up new state funds, based on New York State's Community Mental Health Reinvestment Act of 1993, which mandates that fiscal savings from the closure of state psychiatric hospitals be reinvested into community-based services.[4] This law resulted in the reinvestment of funds in several communities where state hospitals were closed during the George Pataki gubernatorial administration. For example, Westchester County's Department of Community Mental Health received twenty-five million dollars to reinvest in community-based services after the closure of Harlem Valley State Hospital in 1994 (reinvestment dollar amounts would undoubtedly be greater thirty years later).[5] The New York State Office of Mental Health continues to reinvest funds saved when hospital beds are reduced, as documented on its website and in its monthly reports.[6] Funds recouped from the closure of a large state hospital such as Manhattan Psychiatric Center could potentially be used to build new community-based housing with on-site services to support the needs of recently discharged hospital patients who might struggle to live independently (a model known as congregate supportive housing).[7] Funds could also be used to support the rental of apartments in the general community (with off-site supports) to provide permanent housing for shelter residents who are in a position to live more independently (a model known as independent scatter-site housing).

Immediate access to congregate supportive or independent scatter-site housing, in combination with voluntary mental health services, when provided immediately following a stint of homelessness and without requiring preconditions such as abstinence from substances or medication adherence (an approach known as Housing First), has been consistently found to be superior to the delayed "continuum of care" approach that New York currently uses, in which the typical wait time for moving from a shelter to public housing was nearly one year in 2023.[8] In fact, the large multisite At Home/Chez Soi study conducted in five Canadian cities between 2009 and 2013, which randomly assigned more than two thousand homeless individuals with serious mental illnesses to either Housing First or "housing as usual" and followed them up for two years, found that Housing First was associated with better housing stability, improved community participation, and reduced use of costly emergency services.[9] The margin of difference for housing stability was dramatic: the proportion of people assigned to Housing First who were housed "all of the time" over the study period was double that of the treatment-as-usual group. Although Housing First cost $22,257 per person per year, reductions in other costs such as shelters and emergency rooms meant that it was essentially cost neutral. Regarding the effectiveness of congregate supportive or independent scatter-site housing, my own research on the community participation of nearly 350 formerly homeless persons diagnosed with severe mental illnesses in New York City suggests that both forms of housing are effective but that residents of scatter-site housing are able to achieve slightly better community participation than residents of congregate supportive housing.[10] Thus, if institutions on Ward's Island were closed and replaced with a comparable number of units of newly created congregate supportive or independent scatter-site housing, it seems plausible that the creation of new and better-quality supportive housing, located in more central areas of the city, would be a net benefit for Ward's Island's current residents.

If Manhattan Psychiatric Center were closed, most of its patients would likely be transferred to other state hospitals within the New York region. Many within the mental health community do not believe that state psychiatric hospitals are a necessary component of the system and suggest that they should be closed outright. This position is largely linked with the work of the Italian reformer Franco Basaglia, who, beginning in the 1970s, succeeded in creating a movement that led to the closure of all state psychiatric institutions in Italy, replacing them with community-based services.[11] On a recent trip to meet with Italian colleagues, I was told that Basaglia's approach (known as the Trieste Model) is considered a success, and there is no serious consideration of returning to the era of large-scale state hospitalization. However, the Trieste Model has been rejected by most of the Anglophone world and has been minimally considered, if at all, in the United States.[12] It is therefore unlikely that an approach that calls for outright closure and transition to the community of all state hospital patients would succeed within the New York context.

AN ALTERNATE VISION

Another vision for Ward's Island that has recently been articulated by elected officials actually recommends a *reversal* of the nearly seventy-five-year trend toward census reduction at Manhattan Psychiatric Center. Specifically, a report issued in December 2023 by Manhattan Borough President Mark Levine (a Democrat generally regarded as a progressive) called for a "dramatic expansion" at the hospital, increasing its census by four hundred to address the needs of "recently or chronically homeless patients experiencing serious mental illness who would benefit from patient-centered care to prepare for independent living."[13] A census increase of this magnitude would return the census to 550 overall, closer to what it was in the late 1990s.[14] The plan would require renovation of areas of the hospital "which sit entirely vacant" and would therefore potentially require a substantial increase in state funding for this purpose. Readers will recall from the previous chapter that state psychiatric hospitalization is estimated to cost somewhere between one thousand and four thousand dollars per patient per day in New York State (depending on the information source), so the addition of four hundred new state hospital beds would cost between $146 and $584 million per year. For context, the overall annual budget of the New York State Office of Mental Health is $4.5 billion, meaning that this could require a 3–10 percent increase in the agency's annual allocation.[15]

Given the evident high quality of services currently offered at Manhattan Psychiatric Center (as discussed in chapter 7), it is plausible that inpatient treatment would benefit many individuals diagnosed with severe mental illness, and it would certainly be preferable to homelessness. However, given that community-based housing and services are considerably less costly, are preferred by clients over inpatient hospitalization, and are associated with greater life satisfaction and opportunities for community participation, committing such considerable resources to inpatient services can be considered a questionable investment of mental health funding.[16] In contrast to the $1,000–4,000 *per day* cost of hospitalization, rental subsidies generally cover rents of less than $2,000 *per month* in New York City, and the highest level of community-based care, Assertive Community Treatment, costs roughly $2,200 *per month*. The cost of providing both of these services, which is recommended by the Housing First model, would therefore be approximately $50,000 per year, or less than one-seventh the cost of state hospitalization even at the lowest cost estimate of $1,000 per day.

Why would an elected official who has also supported bail reform and other initiatives to reduce the incarceration of people charged with minor crimes recommend the increased involuntary hospitalization of society's most marginalized (predominantly people of color)?[17] Such a perspective is consistent with many of the current statements of Democratic elected officials (as well as their Republican colleagues) who have joined the chorus calling for expanded institutionalization as a response to public outrage over violent crime that is perceived to be related to mental illness.[18] These statements have been influenced by the *New York Times*, which has made a point of calling for greater institutionalization from its editorial page platform and has released a series of special reports suggesting that the failure to involuntarily hospitalize people with mental illness played a direct role in high-profile incidents of violence by people with reported psychiatric histories.[19] The newspaper drew an explicit connection between its reporting and Borough President Levine's call, stating that he "unveiled his plan in the wake of a *New York Times* investigation."[20]

Although not specifically calling for an increase in beds at Manhattan Psychiatric Center, other elected officials or public figures associated with the Democratic Party have made similar statements calling for increased involuntary hospitalization. For example, when speaking at a debate of Democratic candidates for mayor of New York City, candidate Andrew Yang leaned into the narrative of "us vs. them" in calling for institutionalization: "*We* [emphasis added] need to get *them* [emphasis added] off of *our* streets and *our* subways into a better environment. . . . Yes, the mentally ill have rights, but you know who else has rights? *We* do. The people and families of the city."[21] Similarly, speaking at a vigil for a victim of a possible anti-Asian hate crime incident, New York State's attorney general Letitia James directed blame at people with mental illness and the mental health system, stating "we have people living on the street who are a danger to themselves or others—not all people who are struggling with a mental illness are dangerous, but let's be honest, some are. And it's time to say enough. . . . New York State dumped millions of individuals onto our streets with no care."[22]

Aside from being factually inaccurate in multiple ways (e.g., the total decline in the New York state hospital population during the twenty-year height of deinstitutionalization was roughly sixty thousand, nowhere near "millions"),[23] such statements promote the most prominent and damaging of negative stereotypes about people with serious mental illness—that they are dangerous and incapable of living in the community. National surveys indicate that endorsement of these types of negative stereotypes has increased in the general U.S. public in the past decade such that 70 percent of Americans expect that a hypothetical person with schizophrenia is likely to be violent.[24] Further, and alarmingly, research has drawn a clear connection between endorsement of these negative stereotypes and both social avoidance (including unwillingness to have a person with a mental illness as a neighbor, friend, or coworker) and support for more coercive intervention practices, such as involuntary hospitalization.[25] This was articulated by a 2024 *New York Times* letter writer, who stated the position bluntly: "Bring back mental asylums and lock people up who are incapable of functioning in society; it's that simple." More distally, concern about others' endorsement of these negative stereotypes facilitates exactly the type of treatment avoidance that proponents of this perspective claim needs to be responded to with coercive approaches.[26]

Stigma toward people who are homeless can be even more pronounced, with the public showing more fear toward people who are homeless when it intersects with being Black and having a serious mental illness.[27] The extent to which members of the public feel open disdain for people who are homeless can be seen in the way it has been discussed on the social media platform Twitter (now X). In an analysis of all Twitter posts regarding homelessness in the United States over a three-month period in 2013, researchers from the University of California, San Francisco found that posters attributed undesirable characteristics to people who were homeless, suggesting that they were to blame for their situation.[28] Further, disparaging jokes were frequently made, sometimes even trivializing or joking about anti-homeless hate crimes. These findings suggest that stigma toward people with mental illness is likely to be more pronounced when it is combined with homelessness.

Although the reasons for the increased support for negative stereotypes, even among self-identified progressives, are unclear, my colleagues and I have speculated that they have been influenced by the implementation of a successful pro-stigma campaign by groups such as the National Rifle Association and related messaging by other advocacy organizations. These groups have advanced key talking points that have influenced media reports and been echoed by a number of elected officials—"that people with mental illness are subhuman 'monsters,' and the mental health system fails in its responsibility to protect the U.S. public from said 'monsters'"[29] As articulated by the conservative policy analyst Stephen Eide, this position is described as an "anti-anti-stigma" stance, emphasizing "the link between violence and untreated serious mental illness" and "the fact that inpatient psychiatric care is sometimes the best option."[30] Although Democratic Party elected officials and "liberal" media such as the *New York Times* may not use terms like "monsters" and are more likely to use the language of care and concern when discussing mental illness, their emphasis on both dangerousness and the need for coercive treatment show that this anti-anti-stigma campaign has been successful.

In addition to being driven by community stigma, another inherent problem with some of the current discourse around state hospitals is that it presents state hospitalization as a cure for homelessness. This ignores the reality that state hospitalization can sometimes *lead* to homelessness when someone's hospitalization causes them to lose community-based housing that they already have. This is what happened to Carlos, whom I talked about in chapter 1, and it also happened to Linda Andre, a published author and prominent figure in the "psychiatric survivor" movement.[31] Andre experienced lengthy hospitalizations at Manhattan Psychiatric Center between 2015 and 2017, which resulted in her being evicted from a "two-bedroom . . . apartment, a . . . co-op that she owned." As a result, upon discharge from the hospital, she lived on Ward's Island at the transitional living residence (TLR), where she remained until her death, by suicide, in September 2023.[32] Andre's story illustrates just one instance of how state hospitalization can sometimes be a factor in increasing homelessness.

The currently prominent discourse that emphasizes violence among people diagnosed with serious mental illness and presents involuntary hospitalization as a solution to homelessness can certainly be expected to encourage the public to want to continue to "keep people away." From this perspective, it seems unlikely that elected officials would approve the relocation of services from Ward's Island to more central parts of New York City, even given pressure from organizations like RISF/RIPA. If this is the case, then we might expect the siting of services on Ward's Island to only continue to grow.

PROPOSAL FOR A THIRD WAY

Is there another way, one motivated by neither greed (which some might consider to be the motive underlying gentrification) nor fear? Is there a way that instead employs evidence-based approaches to promote socially just outcomes and centers the interests of the people who actually live on Ward's Island (as well as the overall New York City community, which indirectly benefits from improving the lives of its most marginalized)?

When I started working on this book, I was fairly certain that the only way to move forward was to stop locating services in a remote place like Ward's Island, but after conducting interviews with current residents and former staff, I have come to change my position. As readers will recall from the findings presented in the previous chapter, despite their many complaints about the lack of resources and disconnection of living on Ward's Island, many current residents also indicated that they enjoyed its park space and that its location provided them with "comfort and peace." Similarly, as presented earlier in this chapter, former staff members were vehemently opposed to the closure of facilities on the island. This led me to think about whether there might be a way to address the current injustices of life on Ward's Island and honor the idea that the marginalized people currently living there have a right to live there in a dignified way. I considered extensively what could be done and also consulted the urban planning literature for guidance.[33] I also considered the suggestions of the former staff I interviewed, who unanimously and enthusiastically agreed with the idea of providing permanent housing on the island but raised concerns about how feasible it would be without the creation of a parallel infrastructure of services and adequate public transportation.[34] Finally, I spoke with two additional experts: the director of housing services for a large New York–based mental health service agency and the codeveloper of an organization focused on mental health museum exhibits.[35]

What I propose would not lead to the loss of any park space and might provide some area for additional parkland development. My proposal is as follows:

1. Close two of the three large buildings currently used to house Manhattan Psychiatric Center and Kirby Forensic Psychiatric Center and consolidate both hospitals into a single building. Each building was originally created to house 1,000 patients, yet the total number of patients currently housed in all three is only 350. There should therefore be ample

space in a single building to colocate both institutions, meaning that the current use of all three buildings is a waste of valuable and needed space. The most likely candidate for the single hospital building would be the Kirby Building, since adding the various security components that it includes to one of the other buildings would likely be costly. There would be no reduction in state hospital beds as a result of this consolidation, and there would even be room for a small census increase if deemed necessary by policymakers.

2. Rededicate funds from the downsizing of the Manhattan Psychiatric Center/Kirby Forensic campus to reinvestment in new community-based housing and support services on Ward's Island (see below). The reinvestment funds would be used specifically to support subsidized rents for formerly homeless residents who are recipients of Supplemental Security Income and cannot afford to pay market-rate rents.

3. Demolish the two remaining hospital buildings and use the recovered space to construct new permanent housing. Reclaiming this area, as well as associated spaces that would no longer be needed (such as the current hospital "yards" and associated staff parking spaces), can create enough space to develop roughly 1,200 new units of high-quality housing (each unit would essentially be an apartment with its own bathroom and kitchen). As explained to me by the director of a major supportive housing agency in New York City, the model that appears to be most viable would be "mixed-population" housing, allowing for the construction of buildings with a 60–40 percent split between supportive housing for people with serious mental illness and affordable housing for low-income community members. This model enables nonprofit agencies to build by giving them access to federal low-income housing tax credits.[36]

Based on this model, 500 units could be dedicated to permanently house all individuals currently living in both the Keener and Clarke Thomas shelters, in addition to another 220 currently homeless people or marginally housed individuals with serious mental illness from other locations, with preference being given to those who have recently been discharged from Manhattan Psychiatric Center or who recently lived in another setting on Ward's Island. An additional 480 low-income New

Yorkers could be housed in the other 40 percent of units. The area that would be recovered from the demolition of parts of the current Manhattan Psychiatric Center campus is equivalent to roughly sixteen acres, or about the size of three New York City blocks. The average population of a single city block in Manhattan is 1,400, so the area could accommodate the construction of multiple low-density structures comprising at least 1,200 units. I recommend a total of 1,200 units given that Ward's Island's population has hovered around this number for the past twenty years or so, so it is assumed that this number of permanent residents would not place an undue burden on the local mental health providers in East Harlem who already serve the needs of current residents. Structures of eight floors could include enough units to house 180 persons (based on comparable buildings in other locations), along with space for staff offices, service provision (such as skills-training groups), and essential amenities (discussed below). With this low-density arrangement, about seven buildings would be needed. The residences would be managed by a nonprofit mental health/housing provider, who would provide on-site staff and security to coordinate services, through a contract with the New York State Office of Mental Health. (There are a number of such providers, who often deal with challenges such as purchasing land or existing buildings to construct new housing, so the management of already constructed residences would be a sought-after arrangement by comparison.) The construction of high-quality permanent supportive housing in place of shelters is consistent with the evidence-based Housing First approach discussed earlier in this chapter that has been championed by policymakers with compelling evidence that homelessness is primarily a problem of lack of affordable housing.[37] The area of Ward's Island where Manhattan Psychiatric Center is currently located is already zoned to allow for the building of medium-density housing, so it would not require rezoning.[38]

Creation of the housing units would require that the fencing that currently separates the area around the Manhattan Psychiatric Center campus from the open green areas of Ward's Island be removed, as these would present a clear barrier to community participation by the permanently housed residents of these new buildings (fencing would remain around the hospital building itself). This would rectify a current injustice that creates a barrier between the island's residents and park users from the general community.

4. Demolish the Clarke Thomas shelter building and use the area to expand park space consistent with the goals of RISF/RIPA. This would allow RIPA to benefit to some extent and use the space to create a new sports field, garden, or playground.

5. Use ground-floor spaces of the newly built structures to create essential services to accommodate the needs of the newly housed residents so that they no longer have to take the M35 bus to meet basic needs. There should be ample space for these services in the newly constructed buildings. Three essential services should be prioritized: (1) a small- to medium-size grocery store (so that residents can purchase food for meal preparation); (2) a drug store/pharmacy (so that residents can purchase other necessary goods, as well as fill prescriptions for medications to address physical and mental health needs); and (3) a coffee shop or diner that serves inexpensive food (providing a place for persons to eat and congregate). Despite their limited resources, these residents would almost all be recipients of federal SNAP benefits, which currently provide $291/month to individuals for the purchase of food, so a grocery store with a "captive" market of 1,200 residents would likely generate hundreds of thousands in income per month.[39] A drug store/pharmacy would have a similarly favorable market and steady income stream, given that most of the island's residents are prescribed multiple medications that are paid for by Medicaid. Additional space could be provided for other businesses that might wish to open on the island at a later date. Because they would be located on public land, these businesses could be constructed with public funds and pay favorable subsidized rents. They would serve not only island residents but also the many island visitors who currently have no place to go for a quick meal or snack or to purchase supplies for a picnic or barbecue.

Residents of the newly created housing facilities would also be given priority for employment at these newly created businesses, following the Italian "social enterprise" model, which has been supported by research findings.[40] I estimate that the creation of these three businesses would provide opportunities for the employment of 75–125 island residents in a range of full- and part-time roles. In addition to providing residents with an opportunity to work, generate income, and improve community functioning (as research with the Italian social enterprise model has shown), employing residents in these businesses would provide a contact-based "anti-stigma" experience for community members who patronize them.

6. Convert the Keener Building, the oldest of the current structures on the island (which would no longer be functioning as a shelter) into a combined museum and library. The building is an architecturally imposing structure that deserves to be preserved in a way that honors the island's history. The museum portion of the building would be dedicated to educating the public about mental illness; it would be managed by a nonprofit organization with an established track record of advocating for people with serious mental illness, such as the National Alliance on Mental Illness–New York City chapter (NAMI-NYC) or the peer-run agency Baltic Street AEH.[41]

Following recommendations from Dr. Paul Piwko of the National Museum of Mental Health Project, the key focal points of optimal mental health museum exhibits should be "experiential, historic, and cultural." Therefore, I propose that the museum should contain historical exhibits providing information about the history of Ward's Island, Manhattan Psychiatric Center/New York City Asylum for the Insane, and related public psychiatric hospitals in New York State, as well as more experiential exhibits that demystify and destigmatize mental health conditions. The stories of famous residents of the hospital, from Scott Joplin to Russell Jones (aka Ol' Dirty Bastard), could be told and honored. Finally, it would include culturally engaging galleries exhibiting artistic works (including painting and multimedia art) by people diagnosed with mental health conditions, providing visitors the opportunity to engage and understand the experiences of such individuals. As recommended by Dr. Piwko, the museum should also provide information about local services (such as Fountain House, NAMI-NYC, and Baltic Street) to help visitors understand how to gain peer and family support and encourage help-seeking. Mental health museum exhibits exist in a number of major locations in the United States, but there is no exhibit of this type in New York City, despite being the home of roughly 150 museums.[42] In a study of an innovative traveling exhibit called "Mental Health: Mind Matters," colleagues and I noted that it has considerable promise as a model for addressing stigma among community members and helping people with mental illness feel understood.[43] Interestingly, Robert Moses also showed a Health Museum in one of his plans for the redevelopment of Ward's Island (see chapter 3, figure 3.4), so creating a museum would be fulfilling part of his original vision. The museum would help bring additional visitors to the island and provide additional opportunities for interaction between general community members and the marginalized people of Ward's Island.[44] This could lead to further reduction of stigma, consistent with the goals of the New York State Office of Mental Health's current strategic plan to combat mental health stigma.[45]

The creation of a small public library branch with a collection focused on mental health would provide an additional resource for members of the Ward's Island community to read books and gain access to services such as computers, the internet, and word processing software. Of course, general community members could also use the branch while visiting the island.

7. Improve the public transportation infrastructure of the island to facilitate community engagement opportunities for residents to visit families and friends, allow families and friends to visit island residents, and give more general community members greater access to the island's park and other resources (including the proposed museum). The most straightforward way to improve the infrastructure, already proposed by a range of stakeholders (under the name Randall's Island Transit), is to increase the frequency of the M35 bus and run additional buses that travel to both the Bronx and Astoria, Queens (both of which are connected with Ward's Island via the Triborough Bridge).[46] This would increase access to the islands for residents, community members, and staff.

In the long run, another improvement to the transportation infrastructure, proposed by the Regional Plan Association, involves the building of a new subway line that would use the tracks that run over the Hellgate Bridge (currently used exclusively by Amtrak and freight rail lines).[47] This proposed train line (called "The Triboro") would link Queens with the Bronx and include a stop on Ward's or Randall's Island (one of many stops on this new rail line). The Metropolitan Transit Authority (MTA) has made a similar proposal, called "Penn Station Access," that includes a plan to run the Metro-North suburban railway between the Bronx, Queens, and Manhattan over the Amtrak Hell Gate Line, which runs directly over Ward's Island.[48] Although the MTA's proposal does not include stops on Ward's or Randall's Island, the development of permanent housing could justify the allocation of funding for the additional station. While creating a rail link to Ward's Island would be more expensive than expanding bus service, it would further facilitate community participation among Ward's Island's new permanent residents, because trains can accommodate larger numbers than buses and can bring residents to New York's central business district in less time.

An additional strategy that could be implemented to improve transportation access would be the expansion of bike share stations on Ward's Island. New York City currently has a large and successful bike share program called Citi Bike.[49] Ward's Island residents could be given subsidized annual memberships to Citi Bike. Although there is currently one docking station on Ward's Island, it would be insufficient to accommodate the needs of residents; it would need to be significantly expanded, by four or five times, depending on how many residents opt in to low-cost membership. Ward's Island currently has an excellent infrastructure of bike lanes, thanks to the efforts of RISF/RIPA, so increasing the availability of low-cost bikes would be a sensible step toward improving transportation options for the island's residents.

In summary, my proposal includes the construction of decent permanent housing that will reduce the New York City single-adult homeless population by 720; the creation of 480 new units of affordable housing for low-income New Yorkers; the creation of amenities that will serve the needs of residents, allow them to have their needs met on the island, and create job opportunities for island residents; the creation of a museum that will honor Ward's Island's history and provide an exhibit that can be used as a vehicle for stigma reduction; no reduction in the current inpatient beds; and a small increase in park space. My proposal is consistent with recent calls from urban planners to use creative ways to increase the supply of affordable housing in New York City (including the current mayoral administration's "City of Yes" proposal).[50] My plan does not call for any change in the status of the Odyssey House facility, which was recently renovated, or the two existing community residences (the TLR and Jewish Board residence). The creation of amenities for island residents, the removal of unjust fencing, and the improvement of public transportation will benefit all of these residents as well.

My proposal does not address housing for the roughly two thousand asylum seekers currently housed on Ward's Island, as it is not known how long the temporary shelter will remain on the island. It is certainly possible that the proposal could be expanded to create larger structures that can accommodate a combination of asylum seekers and current shelter residents, but I will leave that aside at this point given that there are too many open questions about how long the current migrant crisis will persist.

Although many of the steps outlined above may seem radical, they are not unprecedented in the history of the reclamation of areas where marginalized persons have lived. The clearest precedent is that of Roosevelt Island (formerly known as Welfare Island, and Blackwell's Island before that). As discussed in chapter 2, in the 1800s Blackwell's Island was the home of New York's first public asylum, along with the city jail and an almshouse for the homeless poor. After the closure of the island's institutions, the city located two hospitals for people with physical disabilities on it, but it otherwise sat vacant, and there was almost no way to reach it other than a public bus from Queens. In 1969 an ambitious plan was put forth to create twenty thousand units of housing on the island, with five thousand units dedicated to low-income New Yorkers.[51] Other components of the plan included the creation of a promenade and town squares providing amenities, including a public school. Eventually, the plan also included the creation of a targeted form of transportation between the island and Manhattan, a cable car called the Roosevelt Island Tramway. Although the plan struggled and went through many ups and downs, housing was eventually constructed, opened to its first residents in 1975, and regarded as a "resounding success" by 1977.[52] I lived with my family on the island (rechristened Roosevelt Island) between 1980 and 1983, immediately after we left Ward's Island. Although life there was somewhat removed from Manhattan, I was easily able to get to school in Manhattan every day, and the few local stores that were available at the time were adequate to address our immediate needs. Today, Roosevelt Island has roughly eleven thousand residents and even has its own subway stop, so that residents no longer have to rely on the Tramway to get to Manhattan.[53]

It is also not without precedent for the New York State Office of Mental Health to sell or repurpose land on the former campuses of its state hospitals. For example, the large campus of the now-closed Hudson River Psychiatric Center in Dutchess County has been sold to developers to create a mixed-use development of suburban homes and shopping.[54] Plans include the preservation of a historic hospital structure, which will be restored and converted into a conference center.[55]

Obviously, there are differences between these two development projects and what I am proposing, most notably that they involved leasing public land to developers. Although the Roosevelt Island plan involved the creation of affordable housing, it did not create supportive housing specifically geared to people who have experience homelessness. There is no opportunity for profit in the plan that I have outlined, but rather a rededication of resources toward a public good that advances social justice. The current management of the large structures of the Manhattan Psychiatric Center, the Keener shelter and the Clarke Thomas shelter is expensive and does not advance well-being or justice, as was made amply clear in chapter 7. The only saving grace to life in those institutions is the natural beauty of the island. The plan that I propose would increase access to the natural beauty, as well as improve the material conditions of people's lives. Although I am not focused on clinical stability related to mental illness or substance use, it is plausible that being able to meet basic needs on the island would lead to decreased contact with predatory drug dealing around 125th Street and Lexington Avenue, making it easier for residents to reduce harmful substance use. The plan would also benefit the general community outside of Ward's Island's residents. The availability of amenities and improved public transportation would make it easier and more pleasant to visit both Ward's and Randall's Islands. Further, the social enterprise businesses and mental health museum would serve as vehicles for combating community stigma through contact-based experiences. Such a plan would honor the memories of all those who suffered through decades of substandard treatment, as has been documented in this book. It would also finally allow Ward's Island to move on from its role as a place of urban exile to become instead a place of urban sanctuary.

In conclusion, I believe it is time for New York City to come to terms with the way it has been using Ward's Island as a dumping ground for marginalized groups for the past 180 years and to take explicit steps to make amends for its past and current injustices. This would be consistent with the philosophy of "restorative justice," defined as a "process in which all the stakeholders affected by an injustice have the opportunity to discuss the consequences of the injustice and what might be done to put them right."[56] The steps that I propose are only one possible way of making amends, but I believe they would be a clear and decisive step in this direction.

NOTES

1. A STRANGE JUXTAPOSITION

1. Name and key identifying information have been changed.
2. Regarding SSI, see U.S. Social Security Administration, "Spotlight on Continued SSI Benefits for Persons Who Are Temporarily Institutionalized—2024 Edition," https://www.ssa.gov/ssi/spotlights/spot-temp-institution.htm.
3. S. Seitz and S. Miller, *The Other Islands of New York City: A History and Guide*, 2nd ed. (Woodstock, VT: Countryman Press, 2001).
4. The other state psychiatric hospitals within New York City are Bronx Psychiatric Center, Creedmore Psychiatric Center (in Queens), Kingsboro Psychiatric Center (in Brooklyn), and South Beach Psychiatric Center (in Staten Island). In addition, there is Kirby Forensic Psychiatric Center, a state-run hospital for persons charged with crimes and determined to be not competent to stand trial for psychiatric reasons, also located on Ward's Island.
5. See chapter 2 for details on Manhattan State Hospital's census in the late nineteenth and early twentieth centuries.
6. Department of Psychology, Manhattan Psychiatric Center, *Doctoral Internship Program Brochure*, New York State Office of Mental Health, https://omh.ny.gov/omhweb/facilities/mapc/internship/internshipbrochure.pdf.
7. New York State Department of Transportation, "MTA Bridges & Tunnels Hourly Traffic Rates," https://data.ny.gov/Transportation/MTA-Bridges-Tunnels-Hourly-Traffic-Rates-Beginning/qzve-kjga/data.
8. I base this statement on a survey I conducted in late 2022. Recruiting from an online survey platform called Prolific, I surveyed roughly three hundred New York City residents regarding their awareness of Ward's Island. Although 36 percent of respondents indicated that they had heard of the island, only 7 percent were able to

accurately describe it as a place where an active hospital and/or a homeless shelter were located, with many believing it was the former location of a long-abandoned hospital. More detailed findings from this survey are discussed in chapter 7.

9. S. Seitz and S. Miller, *The Other Islands of New York City: A History and Guide*, 3rd ed. (Woodstock, VT: Countryman Press, 2011).
10. Carlos's fears were not without merit. In late 2022, New York mayor Eric Adams announced a plan for the police to involuntarily detain and escort people who looked like they have a mental illness to local psychiatric hospitals. In discussing the types of situations that could lead one to be involuntarily detained, he cited examples of behavior that could be seen as evidence of mental illness that pose no threat to others such as "shadow boxing" and "mumbling to oneself." City of New York, "Transcript: Mayor Eric Adams Delivers Address on Mental Health Crisis in New York City and Holds Q-and-A," November 29, 2022, https://www.nyc.gov/office-of-the-mayor/news/871-22/transcript-mayor-eric-adams-delivers-address-mental-health-crisis-new-york-city-holds.
11. See D. G. Kingdon and D. Turkington, *Cognitive Therapy of Schizophrenia* (New York: Guilford, 2008).
12. NYC Planning, 2020 Census, https://www.nyc.gov/site/planning/planning-level/nyc-population/2020-census.page.
13. N. Casey, "K2, a Potent Drug, Casts a Shadow Over an East Harlem Block," *New York Times*, September 2, 2015, https://www.nytimes.com/2015/09/03/nyregion/k2-a-potent-drug-casts-a-shadow-over-an-east-harlem-block.html.
14. C. Berghofen, *Randall's and Ward's Island, Manhattan: Phase 1a Archeological Assessment Report* (New York: Triborough Bridge and Tunnel Authority, 2001).
15. See S. Horn, *Damnation Island: Poor, Sick, Mad, and Criminal in Nineteenth-Century New York* (New York: Workman, 2018).
16. A. Scull, *Madness in Civilization* (Princeton, NJ: Princeton University Press, 2015).
17. M. Summers, *Madness in the City of Magnificent Intentions: A History of Race and Mental Illness in the Nation's Capital* (New York: Oxford University Press, 2019).
18. J. C. Phelan, B. G. Link, and J. F. Dovidio, "Stigma and Prejudice: One Animal or Two?," *Social Science and Medicine* 67 (2008): 358–367.
19. This is consistent with a modified "terror management theory" perspective that my colleague Joseph DeLuca and I articulated and found empirical support for. Essentially, this theory proposes that viewing those with mental illnesses as "other" and fundamentally different serves a function of protecting people from the fear that they or people like them could develop a mental illness. J. DeLuca and P. T. Yanos, "Managing the Terror of a Dangerous World: Political Attitudes as Predictors of Mental Health Stigma," *International Journal of Social Psychiatry* 62 (2016): 21–30.
20. An anonymous 2019 *New York Times* letter writer encapsulated these types of unspoken views: "In the phrase 'support for a new homeless shelter' let's replace 'homeless' with 'sex offenders,' 'drug addicts' or 'the mentally ill.' Now show of hands, who wants a shelter for any of those groups in their neighborhood? Yeah, that's what I thought, and the truth is these groups are all overwhelmingly represented among the

homeless.... The issues facing all three of these groups not only have incredibly high recidivism rates but also pose a real public safety threat. No amount of do-gooder platitudes will change that." Metropolitan Desk Reader Comments, *New York Times*, June 9, 2019.

21. M. J. Dear and S. M. Taylor, *Not on Our Street: Community Attitudes Toward Mental Health Care* (London: Pion, 1982).
22. J. P. Webster, *The Philadelphia State Hospital at Byberry: A History of Misery and Medicine* (Charleston, SC: History Press, 2013).
23. National Museum of American History, "Center for Restorative History," https://americanhistory.si.edu/about/centers/restorative-history.

2. WARD'S ISLAND: A PLACE WHERE NO ONE WOULD COMPLAIN

1. I focus on recorded history as documented from the beginning of European colonization, fully acknowledging that this is not the beginning of its history, since the area now known as New York City was inhabited by the Lenape people for thousands of years prior to the arrival of Europeans.
2. W. Kelby, *Notes on Ward's Island* (New York Historical Society, 1981).
3. M. Nichols, "Hell Gate: Names of Fear, Fear of Names," Gotham Center for New York City History, August 14, 2012, https://www.gothamcenter.org/blog/hell-gate-names-of-fear-fear-of-names; D. Denton, *A Brief Description of New York: Formerly Called New Netherlands* (London, 1670), available at Libraries at University of Nebraska–Lincoln, Electronic Texts in American Studies, ed. Paul Royster, 2006.
4. "Names of New York: Wards Island," *Newsday* (New York), September 1, 2000.
5. E. S. Rutsch and R. L. Potter, *Stage One Cultural Resource Survey of the Proposed Sludge Storage Lagoon and the Proposed Access Roadway Wards Island Water Pollution Control Plant, New York City* (Boston: Camp Dresser & McKee, 1980).
6. J. F. Richmond, *New York and Its Institutions, 1609–1872* (New York: E. B. Treat, 1872), 554.
7. Commissioners of Emigration, *Rules for the Government of the Emigrant Refuge and Hospital at Ward's Island* (New York: Casper C. Childs Printer, 1850).
8. S. Seitz and S. Miller, *The Other Islands of New York City: A History and Guide*, 2nd ed. (Woodstock, VT: Countryman Press, 2001), 167.
9. H. M. Hurd, W. F. Drewry, R. Dewey, C. W. Pilgrim, and G. A. Blumer, *The Institutional Care of the Insane in the United States and Canada* (Baltimore, MD: Johns Hopkins Press, 1916).
10. Seitz and Miller, *The Other Islands of New York City*, 2nd ed.
11. "The Purchase of Ward's Island: Opinion of Mayor Tiemann—Interesting Proceedings," *New York Times*, February 11, 1858.
12. Readers will note the name Negro Point on the map. The racially offensive name (with unclear origins) was finally changed in 2001 to Scylla Point after advocacy from Parks

Department commissioner Henry Stern. E. Baard, "Neighborhood Report: Ward's Island; Uneasily Invoking an Outdated Past," *New York Times*, July 8, 2001.

13. P. Smith, *A Short Historical Sketch of Ward's Island* (State of New York, Department of Mental Hygiene, 1947).
14. "Some of the inmates paid from five dollars to twelve dollars a week, but this number and the majority were treated free of charge." Hurd et al., *Institutional Care of the Insane*.
15. W. S. Mills, *History of the First Twenty-Five Years of the Ward's Island and Metropolitan Hospital* (New York: Rooney and Otten, 1900).
16. L. Davidson, J. Rakfeldt, and J. Strauss, *The Roots of the Recovery Movement in Psychiatry: Lessons Learned* (Hoboken, NJ: Wiley, 2011).
17. The modern descendent of the Bloomingdale Asylum is located in White Plains, Westchester County, and is part of the New York–Presbyterian Hospital system.
18. F. M. Bixby and D. H. Olmstead, *The Bloomingdale Lunatic Asylum of the City of New York: Why It Should Pay Taxes, Why Its Streets Should Be Opened, Why It Should Be Removed from the City* (New York: Lexington Middlerich Law Printer, 1888).
19. A source indicates that there was a brief period during which the "insane poor" of New York City were treated at Bloomingdale, but this ended in 1825. Hurd et al., *Institutional Care of the Insane*.
20. M. Summers, *Madness in the City of Magnificent Intentions: A History of Race and Mental Illness in the Nation's Capital* (New York: Oxford University Press, 2019).
21. S. Horn, *Damnation Island: Poor, Sick, Mad, and Criminal in Nineteenth-Century New York* (New York: Workman, 2018).
22. Department of Public Charities and Corrections, *Annual Reports of the New York City Asylum for the Insane, Ward's Island, NY, for the Years 1874–1886* (New York: Bellevue Press); Hurd et al., *Institutional Care of the Insane*.
23. "Obituaries: Alexander E. MacDonald, MD," *Boston Medical and Surgery Journal* 155 (1906): 727–728.
24. One building, the Verplanck, was described as "pretentious" by an early twentieth-century source. P. Smith, *A Short Historical Sketch of Ward's Island* (State of New York, Department of Mental Hygiene, 1947). See also C. Yanni, *Architects of Madness: Insane Asylums in the United States* (Minneapolis: University of Minnesota Press, 2007).
25. Inflation-adjustment calculators go back only to 1913 (see https://www.bls.gov/data/inflation_calculator.htm), but if we assume a 1913 scale, then thirty-three cents would be the equivalent of only ten dollars per day in 2023, at least a hundred times less than the current cost of housing patients in the hospital (discussed in chapter 7).
26. Hurd et al., *Institutional Care of the Insane*, 203.
27. Hurd et al., *Institutional Care of the Insane*, 206.
28. J. Henssler, L. Brandt, M. Müller, S. Liu, C. Montag, P. Sterzer, and A. Heinz, "Migration and Schizophrenia: Meta-Analysis and Explanatory Framework," *European Archives of Psychiatry and Clinical Neuroscience* 270 (2020): 325–335, 325.
29. G. Makari, *Of Fear and Strangers: A History of Xenophobia* (New York: Norton, 2021).

30. N. I. Painter, *The History of White People* (New York: Norton, 2010).
31. G. N. Grob, *Mental Institutions in America: Social Policy to 1875* (New York: Free Press, 1973).
32. A. Vadukul, "The Forgotten Entertainer Rag," *New York Times*, May 24, 2018, https://www.nytimes.com/2018/05/24/nyregion/remembering-scott-joplin.html.
33. M. Summers, *Madness in the City of Magnificent Intentions: A History of Race and Mental Illness in the Nation's Capital* (New York: Oxford University Press, 2019).
34. Hurd et al., *Institutional Care of the Insane*.
35. A. Hylton, *Madness: Race and Insanity in a Jim Crow Asylum* (New York: Legacy Lit, 2024); J. M. Galt, "Asylums for Colored Persons," *American Psychological Journal* 1 (1853): 78–88, 85.
36. Summers, *Madness in the City of Magnificent Intentions*.
37. In Galt's words, "Lunatics laboring under dementia, take less notice, as a general rule, of their situation and companions, than those afflicted with the other varieties of insanity."
38. "Murdered by a Manic: Tragedy in the Insane Asylum," *New York Times*, October 15, 1878.
39. "The Ward's Island Asylum: The Recent Outrages—Neglect of the Commissioners," *New York Times*, November 13, 1872.
40. Grob, *Mental Institutions in America*.
41. Alexander E. Macdonald Papers and Photographs, 1865–1906 (New York Academy of Medicine).
42. *Annual Reports of the Managers of the Manhattan State Hospital at New York, NY to the State Commission in Lunacy, 1897–1899* (Albany, NY: Wynkoop Hallenbeck Crawford Co. State Printers); *Annual Reports of the Manhattan State Hospital to the Board of Managers, 1905–1933* (Utica, NY: State Hospital Press).
43. See Government of the City of New York, "Total and Foreign-Born Population New York City, 1790–2000," https://www.nyc.gov/assets/planning/download/pdf/planning-level/nyc-population/historical-population/1790-2000_nyc_total_foreign_birth.pdf.
44. B. Malzberg, *Social and Biological Aspects of Mental Disease* (Utica, NY: State Hospitals Press, 1940).
45. N. Bly, *Ten Days in a Madhouse* (New York: Ian L. Munro, 1887).
46. The report can be found in its entirety within the 1892 annual report.
47. A 1916 source did boast that "Manhattan is the largest and one of the best psychiatrical [sic] hospitals in the world.... Many of its patients never in their lives enjoyed such comforts as they now do," but this conflicts with accounts written by hospital superintendents. Hurd et al., *Institutional Care of the Insane*, 207.
48. D. Penney and P. Stastny, *The Lives They Left Behind: Suitcases from a State Hospital Attic* (New York: Bellevue, 2008).
49. "The Ward's Island Tragedy," *New York Times*, February 20, 1923.
50. S. D. Lamb, *Pathologist of the Mind: Adolf Meyer and the Origins of American Psychiatry* (Baltimore, MD: Johns Hopkins University Press, 2014).

3. PARKLAND OR INSTITUTIONAL DUMPING GROUND?

1. The bridge did provide some indirect opportunities for resourceful individuals to find their way off the island. Harry Hallier, a patient who had served in World War I and was praised for heroically saving the lives of forty other patients during the 1923 fire, subsequently escaped from the hospital by sneaking through a "hollow girder in the Hell Gate Bridge." "Ward's Island Now Expanding—Upward," *New York World Tribune,* March 6, 1954.
2. See W. Donaldson, "First Year's Operation of Wards Island Sewage Treatment Works," *Sewage Works Journal* 11 (1939): 100–116.
3. *Annual Reports of the Manhattan State Hospital to the Board of Managers,* 1928–29, 1935–36, 25–32; 1936–37, 1949–50, 33–46 (Utica, NY: State Hospital Press).
4. See H. Ballon and K. T. Jackson, *Robert Moses and the Modern City: The Transformation of New York* (New York: Norton, 2008).
5. "Ward's Island Bill Signed by Governor," *New York Times,* April 10, 1929.
6. R. A. Caro, *The Power Broker: Robert Moses and the Fall of New York* (New York: Knopf, 1974).
7. S. Seitz and S. Miller, *The Other Islands of New York City: A History and Guide,* 2nd ed. (Woodstock, VT: Countryman Press, 2001).
8. Caro, *The Power Broker.*
9. New York, State Laws of 1933, Chapter 144.
10. Robert Moses Papers, Box 12. New York Public Library.
11. *Annual Reports of the Board of Managers of the Manhattan State Hospital.* I nearly fell out of my chair when I read this statement because, although the fare has increased substantially since 1937, the pickup/drop-off location for the bus and its frequency of service have remained essentially unchanged in the intervening eighty-seven years. A Randall's Island transit site suggests that, for a limited period, buses also ran to Astoria, Queens and parts of the Bronx, but these additional routes were discontinued in the 1980s. I do not recall these buses being available when I lived on the island in the 1970s, and they had been discontinued when I returned to the island as a volunteer in 1989. See https://randallsislandtransit.org/.
12. *Annual Reports of the Board of Managers of the Manhattan State Hospital.*
13. B. Maltzberg, "A Statistical Study of Patients in the New York Civil State Hospitals, April 1, 1947," *Psychiatric Quarterly* 22 (1948): 497–515; "A Statistical Study of Patients in the New York Civil State Hospitals, April 1, 1950," *Psychiatric Quarterly* 26 (1952): 70–85. Pilgrim and Kings Park grew to be the two largest hospitals in the state system partly as a result of these mass transfers, with a combined census of more than 17,000 in 1947 and 21,000 in 1950.
14. "Huge Island Park Planned for City," *New York Times,* May 15, 1934.
15. While the number of admissions of persons with "psychosis" related to cerebrovascular disease and dementia increased, the number of admissions related to syphilis began to decrease. Syphilis eventually disappeared as a cause of admission after penicillin became widely available, but the decline prior to this was likely due to the increased use of condoms as a form of prevention during the 1930s. E. Wuebker,

"Taking the Venereal Out of Venereal Disease: The 1930s Public Health Campaign Against Syphilis and Gonorrhea," *Notches*, May 31, 2016, https://notchesblog.com/2016/05/31/taking-the-venereal-out-of-venereal-disease-the-1930s-public-health-campaign-against-syphilis-and-gonorrhea/.

16. P. T. Yanos, *Written Off: Mental Health Stigma and the Loss of Human Potential* (New York: Cambridge University Press, 2018).
17. B. Malzberg, "Mental Disease Among Native and Foreign-Born Negroes in New York State," *Journal of Negro Education* 25 (1956): 175–181.
18. These elevated rates of dementia praecox contrast with assertions made by Jonathan Metzl, who contends that schizophrenia was a predominantly "white female" diagnostic category in the United States until the late 1960s, when it became "racialized" and associated with Black men. J. M. Metzl, *The Protest Psychosis: How Schizophrenia Became a Black Disease* (Boston: Beacon Press, 2009). Malzberg's data suggest that, at least in New York State, schizophrenia was disproportionately diagnosed among Black individuals in the early part of the twentieth century. Note that *The Protest Psychosis* primarily draws on records from a state psychiatric hospital in Michigan, where patterns may have differed from New York.
19. D. M. Anglin, S. Ereshefsky, M. J. Klaunig, M. A. Bridgwater, T. A. Niendam, L. M. Ellman, et al., "From Womb to Neighborhood: A Racial Analysis of Social Determinants of Psychosis in the United States," *American Journal of Psychiatry* 178, no. 7 (2021): 599–610, 599.
20. J. A. Lieberman, *Shrinks: The Untold Story of Psychiatry* (New York: Back Bay, 2015).
21. Alcoholics Anonymous was founded as an organization of mutual support to maintain abstinence from alcohol in 1935 in Akron, Ohio by William Wilson (a New Yorker traveling on business) and Robert Smith, a surgeon. See Alcoholics Anonymous, "History of A.A.," https://www.aa.org/aa-history.
22. "Proceedings, Conference of the New York State Commission to Formulate a Long Range Health Program to Consider Problems Arising Through the Proposed Demolition of Manhattan State Hospital on Ward's Island," New York, February 7, 1941, unpublished manuscript, New York City Municipal Archives.
23. *Annual Reports of the Board of Managers of the Manhattan State Hospital.*
24. A. Deutsch, *The Shame of the States* (New York: Harcourt Brace, 1948), 66, 69, 70.
25. Robert Moses Papers, Box 12, New York Public Library.

4. THE *FRENCH CONNECTION* CONNECTION

1. "Ward's Island Bill Signed: City Permitted to Lease Land for Hospital to State," *New York Times*, March 12, 1952.
2. "Wards Island Now Expanding—Upward: Three Skyscrapers Will House State Hospital for Mentally Sick," *New York World Telegram*, March 6, 1954.
3. *Annual Report of the Board of Managers of the Manhattan State Hospital to the State Hospital Commission*, 1950–51 to 1960–61 (Utica, NY: State Hospital Press), 47–57.

4. "Ward's Island," *New York Times*, March 26, 1951.
5. "Ward's Island Footbridge and Park Open: Moses Calls 'Planning Experts' No Help," *New York Times*, May 19, 1951.
6. "Ward's Island," *New York Times*, July 13, 1954; J. C. Ingram, "Big Park Ignored, Despite Beauties: Ward's Island Attracts Fewer Than 1,000 Sunday Visitors for Baseball and Picnics," *New York Times*, July 12, 1954.
7. T. A. Ban, "Fifty Years Chlorpromazine: A Historical Perspective," *Neuropsychiatric Disease and Treatment* 3 (2007): 495–500.
8. *Annual Report of the Board of Managers of the Manhattan State Hospital*, 1950–51 to 1960–61, 47–57.
9. H. Brill and R. E. Patton, "Analysis of State Hospital Reduction in New York State's Mental Hospitals During the First Four Years of Large-Scale Therapy with Psychotropic Drugs," *American Journal of Psychiatry* 116 (1959): 495–509.
10. H. C. B. Denber, "Group Process in a State Hospital," *American Journal of Orthopsychiatry* 33, no. 5 (1963): 900–911, 903.
11. R. C. Hunter and H. M. Forstenzer, "The New York State Community Mental Health Services Act: Its Birth and Early Development," *American Journal of Psychiatry* 113 (1957): 680–685.
12. H. Brill and R. E. Patton, "Analysis of 1955–1956 Population Fall in New York State Mental Hospital in the First Year of Large-Scale Use of Tranquilizing Drugs," *American Journal of Psychiatry* 114 (1957): 509–517.
13. G. N. Grob, *The Mad Among Us: A History of Care of America's Mentally Ill* (New York: Free Press, 1994).
14. A. Deutsch, *The Shame of the State* (New York: Harcourt Brace, 1948).
15. Joint Commission on Mental Illness and Health, *Action for Mental Health* (New York: Basic Books, 1961).
16. My attempt to gain access to subsequent reports by way of a Freedom of Information request resulted in a denial, indicating that the reports, if they existed, had been moved to a remote storage facility and retrieving them would constitute a "herculean or unreasonable" effort.
17. M. Schumach, "A Pervasive Fear Stalks Wards I. Mental Centers," *New York Times*, October 20, 1974.
18. S. Pinker, *The Better Angels of Our Nature: Why Violence Has Declined* (New York: Viking, 2011).
19. See "New York Crime Rates 1960–2019," https://www.disastercenter.com/crime/nycrime.htm.
20. T. J. English, *The Savage City: Race, Murder and a Generation on Edge* (New York: William Morrow, 2011).
21. J. Gfroerer and M. Brodsky, "The Incidence of Illicit Drug Use in the United States, 1962–1989," *British Journal of Addiction* 87 (1992): 1345–1351.
22. "Waiting for the Man," released in 1967 but written by Lou Reed several years earlier, opens with the lines: "I'm waiting for my man / got 26 dollars in my hand / Up to

Lexington 125 / Feel sick and dirty more dead than alive." Although a cover version performed by David Bowie indicated that he misunderstood the song as referencing a sexual encounter, Reed had always been clear that "the man" referred to a drug seller. W. Hermes, *Lou Reed: The King of New York* (New York: Farrar, Strauss & Giroux, 2023).

23. J. M. Metzl, *The Protest Psychosis: How Schizophrenia Became a Black Disease* (Boston: Beacon Press, 2009).
24. During this period New York City also experienced a fiscal crisis, which may have indirectly affected state funding for mental health services because part of the "rescue plan" for the city involved the state's taking over fiscal responsibility for running the City University of New York (a large system of colleges and my employer) in 1976. K. Phillips-Fein, "The Legacy of the 1970s Fiscal Crisis," *Nation*, April 16, 2013, https://www.thenation.com/article/archive/legacy-1970s-fiscal-crisis/.
25. G. Spagnoli, "State to Consolidate Mental Health Units," *New York Daily News*, April 26, 1976.
26. M. Breasted, "Psychiatric Unit on Ward's Island Rebuts Sharp Criticism by Levitt," *New York Times*, February 26, 1977.
27. R. Sullivan, "Sculpture Pieces Enliven Grounds of Mental Center on Wards I," *New York Times*, October 24, 1977.
28. J. Perrault, "Pleasure Island," *Soho News*, July 1, 1981.
29. G. Koz, *Made in South Africa: A Psychiatrist's Journey* (Petersburg, VA: Dietz Press, 2021).
30. G. Koz, "Catch-22: The Psychiatrist in the State Hospital," *Psychiatric Annals* 9 (1979): 47–54, 54.
31. D. Gentle, "Mental Hospital Staff Hike Called 'a Joke,'" *New York Daily News*, June 15, 1980.
32. Grob, *The Mad Among Us*.
33. A. S. Weinstein and M. Cohen, "Young Chronic Patients and Changes in the State Hospital Population," *Hospital and Community Psychiatry* 35 (1984): 595–600.
34. A. Elison, "Average Hospital Expenses Per Inpatient Day Across 50 States," *Becker Hospital Review*, 2020, https://www.beckershospitalreview.com/finance/average-hospital-expenses-per-inpatient-day-across-50-states-02282020.html.
35. Koz, "Catch-22." Dr. MacDonald had reported, "There is not a town or village upon this continent that spends as little upon its Insane as this great City of New York." *Annual Reports of the Managers of the Manhattan State Hospital at New York, NY to the State Commission in Lunacy, 1897–1899* (Albany, NY: Wynkoop Hallenbeck Crawford).
36. J. Sibley, "Child Mental Unit to Be Built Here: Clearing of a Site on Ward's Island Begun by Rockefeller," *New York Times*, November 16, 1965.
37. P. Kihs, "State's Mentally Ill Children Neglected, Civic Group Charges," *New York Times*, April 27, 1970.
38. New York State Commission on Quality of Care for the Mentally Disabled, *Manhattan Children's Psychiatric Center: A Review of Living Conditions*, 1987.

39. S. Gabel, A. J. Swanson, and R. Schindledecker, "Outcome in Children's Day Treatment: Relationship to Preadmission Variables," *International Journal of Partial Hospitalization* 6 (1990): 129–137.
40. M. Schumach, "Hospital Better Than Willowbrook, and Yet . . .," *New York Times*, August 24, 1974.
41. B. Weiser, "Beatings, Burns, and Betrayals: The Willowbrook School's Legacy," *New York Times*, February 21, 2020.
42. M. Schumach, "Retardates Moved to Wards I. Now Victims of Overcrowding," *New York Times*, November 2, 1974. (Note the use of terms, here and below, that are now considered offensive.)
43. L. Miflin and H. Wyatt, "Gas-Periled Shelter Gets Okay," *New York Daily News*, December 4, 1974; "Difficulty Reported Relocating Retarded Patients at Closing Unit," *New York Times*, September 14, 1977.
44. B. Walker, "Odyssey House Inc. of New York," *Journal of Substance Abuse Treatment* 5 (1988): 113–115.
45. P. Benjamin, "Widespread Debris Indicates Neglect at Manhattan's Only Park with Picnic Grounds," *New York Times*, July 20, 1963.
46. H. Ballon and K. T. Jackson, *Robert Moses and the Modern City: The Transformation of New York* (New York: Norton, 2008).

5. "IN ACCORDANCE WITH THE STANDARDS"

1. K. Hopper, *Reckoning with Homelessness* (Ithaca, NY: Cornell University Press, 2003). In full disclosure, Dr. Hopper was a mentor to me earlier in my career.
2. There is still a men's shelter at that location. There is also a five-star hotel next door.
3. See Coalition for the Homeless, "Why Are So Many People Homeless?," https://www.coalitionforthehomeless.org/why-are-so-many-people-homeless/.
4. See Coalition for the Homeless, "Why Are So Many People Homeless?"
5. R. Reich and L. Siegel, "The Emergence of the Bowery as a Psychiatric Dumping Ground," *Psychiatric Quarterly* 50 (1978): 191–201.
6. K. Hopper, "More Than Passing Strange: Homelessness and Mental Illness in New York City," *American Ethnologist* 15 (1988): 155–167.
7. C. Kaiser, "A State Judge Orders Creation of 750 Beds for Bowery Homeless," *New York Times*, December 9, 1979; see also Coalition for the Homeless, "Why Are So Many People Homeless?"
8. G. Koz, *Made in South Africa: A Psychiatrist's Journey* (Petersburg, VA: Dietz Press, 2021).
9. Lluís Alexandre Casanovas Blanco, "A Cut Above the Streets: Robert M. Hayes, Co-Founder of Coalition for the Homeless, in Conversation with Lluís Alexandre Casanovas Blanco," Archinect, May 1, 2019, https://archinect.com/features/article/150133042/a-cut-above-the-streets-robert-m-hayes-co-founder-of-coalition-for-the-homeless-in-conversation-with-llu-s-alexandre-casanovas-blanco.

5. "IN ACCORDANCE WITH THE STANDARDS"

10. I do not have any personal memories of the opening of the shelter on Ward's Island, but it is probably not a coincidence that my family decided to move off the island at around this time, in the summer of 1980.
11. G. Fowler, "Koch Pays Visit to New Shelter on Ward's Island," *New York Times*, January 4, 1980.
12. B. Herbert, "City Shelters Homeless in Their Cold War: Wards Isle Praised Warmly," *New York Daily News*, January 4, 1980.
13. R. Herman, "New York City Resists State on Shelter for Homeless in Residential Areas," *New York Times*, December 30, 1980.
14. M. Kramer and B. Kates, "OK 400-Bed Addition for City's Homeless Men," *New York Daily News*, June 13, 1981.
15. R. Herman, "Hospital Group on Wards I. Sues to Close Men's Shelter," *New York Times*, October 8, 1981.
16. Coalition for the Homeless, *The Callahan Consent Decree Establishing a Legal Right to Shelter for Homeless Individuals in New York City*, https://www.coalitionforthehomeless.org/wp-content/uploads/2014/06/CallahanConsentDecree.pdf.
17. E. G. Fitzsimmons, "New York City Moves to Suspend Right-to-Shelter Mandate," *New York Times*, October 4, 2023.
18. P. Kihss, "Influx of Former Mental Patients Burdening City, Albany Is Told," *New York Times*, November 23, 1980.
19. R. Herman, "New York City Resists State on Shelter for Homeless in Residential Areas," *New York Times*, December 30, 1980.
20. Coalition for the Homeless, "Why Are So Many People Homeless?"; B. Sullivan and J. Burke, "Single-Room Occupancy Housing in New York City: The Origins and Dimensions of a Crisis," *CUNY Law Review* 17 (2014): 901–931; Hopper, "More Than Passing Strange."
21. Social Security, "SSI Federal Payment Amounts," https://www.ssa.gov/OACT/COLA/SSIamts.html; Elika Insider, "Analyzing 100 Years of Real Estate Price History in Manhattan," https://www.elikarealestate.com/blog/tracing-buying-real-estate-new-york-past-100-years/.
22. These are averages; more affordable rents were of course available. For example, the first apartment that I rented with a roommate in 1992, a spacious two-bedroom, cost nine hundred dollars per month, considerably lower than the average rent for the 1980s.
23. Hopper, "More Than Passing Strange," 162.
24. G. Colburn and C. P. Aldern, *Homelessness Is a Housing Problem: How Structural Factors Explain U.S. Patterns* (Oakland: University of California Press, 2023), 10.
25. R. Herman, "New York City Psychiatric Wards Overflow as State Changes Its Mental Health Role," *New York Times*, December 8, 1980.
26. P. F. Eagle and C. Caton, "Homelessness and Mental Illness," in *Homeless in America*, ed. C. Caton (New York: Oxford University Press, 1990).
27. B. Pepper, M. C. Kirschner, and H. Ryglewicz, "The Young Adult Chronic Patient: Overview of a Population," *Hospital and Community Psychiatry* 32 (1981): 463–469.

28. A. S. Weinstein and M. Cohen, "Young Adult Chronic Patients and Changes in the State Hospital Population. *Hospital and Community Psychiatry* 35 (1984): 595–600.
29. Hopper, "More Than Passing Strange."
30. E. R. Shipp, "Suit on Homeless Mental Patients Asks New York State for Housing," *New York Times*, May 21, 1982.
31. J. Barbanell, "Lawsuits Fault the Discharge of Mentally Ill," *New York Times*, October 28, 1987.
32. Koz, *Made in South Africa*.
33. M. S. Kearney, B. H. Harris, F. Jácome, and L. Parker *Ten Economic Facts About Crime and Incarceration in the United States*, The Hamilton Project, May 2014, https://www.brookings.edu/wp-content/uploads/2016/06/v8_THP_10CrimeFacts.pdf. Note that the War on Drugs can also be understood to largely account for the overrepresentation of people diagnosed with serious mental illnesses in jails and prisons in the United States. While deinstitutionalization is often invoked as an explanation for this, it is impossible to discount the impact of the War on Drugs and the parallel rise of mass incarceration. W. H. Fisher, E. Silver, and N. Wolff, "Beyond Criminalization: Toward a Criminologically Informed Framework for Mental Health Policy and Services Research," *Administration and Policy in Mental Health and Mental Health Services Research* 33 (2006): 544–557.
34. M. Alexander, *The New Jim Crow: Mass Incarceration in the Age of Colorblindness* (New York: New Press, 2010).
35. Coalition for the Homeless, "Why Are So Many People Homeless?"
36. Coalition for the Homeless, "Why Are So Many People Homeless?"
37. Colburn and Aldern, *Homelessness Is a Housing Problem*.
38. U.S. Department of Housing and Urban Development, "HUD 2022 Continuum of Care Homeless Assistance Programs Homeless Populations and Subpopulations," https://files.hudexchange.info/reports/published/CoC_PopSub_NatlTerrDC_2022.pdf.
39. S. Seitz and S. Miller, *The Other Islands of New York City: A History and Guide*, 2nd ed. (Woodstock, VT: Countryman Press, 2001).
40. G. Pirelli and P. A. Zapf, "An Attempted Meta-Analysis of the Competency Restoration Research: Important Findings for Future Directions," *Journal of Forensic Psychology Research and Practice* 20 (2020): 134–162; M. McClelland, "When 'Not Guilty' Is a Life Sentence," *New York Times*, September 27, 2017, https://www.nytimes.com/2017/09/27/magazine/when-not-guilty-is-a-life-sentence.html.
41. R. Sullivan, "New Hospital for Criminally Insane Gets No Funds," *New York Times*, January 22, 1984.
42. R. C. Wack, "Forensic Treatment in the United States: A Survey of Selected Forensic Hospital Treatment Services at Kirby Forensic Psychiatric Center," *International Journal of Law and Psychiatry* 16 (1993): 83–104.
43. Koz, *Made in South Africa*.
44. B. English and M. A. Giordano, "Bedlam in Mental Health: The Community Solution," *New York Daily News*, December 14, 1982.

45. J. Ferman and S. E. Katz, "Public Psychiatry: The Road to Revitalization," *Psychiatric Quarterly* 57 (1985): 173–181.
46. R. Smothers, "The Death of a Psychiatric Patient: The Grey Area of Restraint," *New York Times*, February 17, 1982.
47. New York State Commission on Quality of Care for the Mentally Disabled, *Manhattan Psychiatric Center: A Review of Living Conditions*, 1986.
48. W. A. Anthony and R. P. Liberman, "The Practice of Psychiatric Rehabilitation: Historical, Conceptual, and Research Base," *Schizophrenia Bulletin* 12 (1986): 542–559.
49. "Man, 35, Is Hacked to Death on Wards I," *New York Daily News*, November 2, 1990; D. Lorch, "Five Arrested in Halloween Attack on Homeless Men," *New York Times*, November 5, 1900.
50. J. A. McKinley, "Wilding Youth and Homeless: A Blood Feud," *New York Times*, November 3, 1990.
51. National Coalition for the Homeless, *20 Years of Hate*, December 2020, https://nationalhomeless.org/wp-content/uploads/2020/12/hate-crimes-2018-2019_web.pdf.
52. "Anticrime Tactic: Shut Footbridge," *New York Times*, November 13, 1994.

6. WHERE WILL THESE CHILDREN PLAY?

1. New York City Mayor's Office of Criminal Justice, "Fact Sheet: 2020 Shootings and Murders," https://criminaljustice.cityofnewyork.us/wp-content/uploads/2021/01/2020-Shootings-and-Murder-factsheet_January-2021.pdf.
2. R. W. Snyder, *Crossing Broadway: Washington Heights and the Promise of New York City* (Ithaca, NY: Cornell University Press, 2015).
3. Although low-income communities of color were targeted by police, research evidence suggests that users of illegal drugs were (and are) more likely to be white. I felt this keenly in 1992–1994 when I lived in on the border between Morningside Heights (where Columbia University is located) and the lower-income Manhattan Valley, where drug sellers vied to reach the profitable college student market.
4. New cases of HIV rose to 12,719 in 1993, and annual deaths due to HIV rose to 8,345 in 1994; both have declined steadily since then. The earliest waves of the epidemic directly affected the Manhattan Psychiatric Center community, as two of its lead psychiatrists (Roger Biron and Yves Chenier) died in the early 1980s of what became known as AIDS. I recall how upset my father was as his colleagues rapidly became ill; this was my first awareness of the existence of AIDS. Dr. Koz also discusses the passing of these psychiatrists in his autobiography. For details on New York's HIV case and death trends, see NYC Department of Health and Mental Hygiene, New York City HIV/AIDS Annual Surveillance Statistics 2014, https://www.nyc.gov/assets/doh/downloads/pdf/ah/surveillance2014-trend-tables.pdf.
5. P. Stevenson, "Hide the Goal Posts: Girls Are Coming! Buckley vs. Brearly: A Turf War Over Turf," *New York Observer*, October 4, 1993. In full disclosure, I attended a

different all-boys private school in the early to mid-1980s but didn't play any sports, so I have no recollection of whether that school was a participant in the use of fields on Ward's Island.

6. D. Martin, "Plan Takes Shape for a Randall's Island City Recreation Center," *New York Times*, July 18, 1994.
7. S. Seitz and S. Miller, *The Other Islands of New York City: A History and Guide*, 3rd ed. (Woodstock VT: Countryman Press, 2011).
8. Martin, "Plan Takes Shape"; D. L. Lewis, "City 20m Sport for Randalls Is.," *New York Daily News*, May 27, 1993.
9. Some suggestions of conflict of interest in the dual appointment were raised by New York City's comptroller in a 2011 audit, which noted that Aimee Boden received salary supplements from RISF that were not clearly communicated with the Conflict of Interest Board. The audit, though not finding evidence of wrongdoing, recommended that "compensation to City employees from private entities requires tighter controls." City of New York, Office of the Comptroller, *Audit Report on the Randall's Island Sports Foundation's Compliance with Its License Agreement with the City of New York Department of Parks and Recreation*, 2011.
10. Randall's Island Park Alliance, "Rudy Bruner Award for Urban Excellence Application," 2005.
11. Office of the Mayor, Rudolph Giuliani, "Randall's Island: Requests for Expressions of Interest," 1999.
12. New York City Department of Parks & Recreation, Wards Island Park, https://www.nycgovparks.org/parks/wards-island-park/history; Randall's Island Park Alliance, Park Map, https://randallsisland.org/wp-content/uploads/2024/01/RIPA-MAP-2023.pdf.
13. N. M. Davidson and D. Fagundes, "Law and Neighborhood Names," *Vanderbilt Law Review* 72 (2019): 757–824.
14. G. Lakoff, *The Political Mind: A Cognitive Scientist's Guide to Your Brain and Its Politics* (New York: Penguin, 2008).
15. As local blogger Led Black put it: "Simply stated Hudson Heights doesn't exist. It was created to appeal to non-locals because Washington Heights had a certain stigma to it." Led Black, "Op-Led: Hudson Heights Doesn't Exist," Uptown Collective, April 6, 2018, https://www.uptowncollective.com/2018/04/06/op-led-hudson-heights-doesnt-exist/.
16. L. Freeman and F. Braconi, "Gentrification and Displacement New York City in the 1990s," *Journal of the American Planning Association* 70, no. 1 (2004): 39–52.
17. I. Anguelovski, J. J. Connolly, H. Cole, M. Garcia-Lamarca, M. Triguero-Mas, F. Baró, et al., "Green Gentrification in European and North American Cities," *Nature Communications* 13, no. 1 (2022): 3816.
18. S. Seitz and S. Miller, *The Other Islands of New York City: A History and Guide*, 2nd ed. (Woodstock VT: Countryman Press, 2001); 3rd ed. (Woodstock VT: Countryman Press, 2011), 195.
19. Stevenson, "Hide the Goal Posts."

20. Seitz and Miller, *The Other Islands of New York City*, 3rd ed., 188.
21. P. T. Yanos, *Written Off: Mental Health Stigma and the Loss of Human Potential*. (New York: Cambridge University Press, 2018).
22. New York City Mayor's Office of Criminal Justice, "Fact Sheet: 2020 Shootings and Murders."
23. Office of the Mayor, "Randall's Island: Requests for Expressions of Interest."
24. E. Badger and L. Ferre-Sadurni, "As Bloomberg's New York Prospered, Inequality Flourished Too," *New York Times*, November 9, 2019.
25. Seitz and Miller, *The Other Islands of New York City*, 3rd ed., 180.
26. Randall's Island Park Alliance, Park Map.
27. D. Feiden, "Footbridge Is Span-Tastic," *New York Daily News*, June 1, 2012.
28. Randall's Island Park Alliance, *Review 2013–2014*, 2014, https://docslib.org/doc/637871/review-2013-2014-dear-friend-of-randall-s-island-park.
29. T. Williams, "On Randalls Island, New Ball Fields via Deal with Elite Schools," *New York Times*, February 10, 2007; A. Hartocolis, "Judge Queries Plan to Give Private Schools Priority on Randalls Island," *New York Times*, January 11, 2008.
30. J. Anderson, "On Randalls Island, Private Schools Play Free," *New York Times*, June 13, 2010.
31. Seitz and Miller, *The Other Islands of New York City*, 3rd ed., 194.
32. Coalition for the Homeless, "Why Are So Many People Homeless?," https://www.coalitionforthehomeless.org/why-are-so-many-people-homeless/#1990-1993.
33. One report found that misdemeanor arrest rates of Black New Yorkers nearly doubled during the 1990s, going from roughly 4.5 per hundred thousand in 1990 to roughly 8.5 per hundred thousand in 2000. I encountered the effects of this in the late 1990s at the Riker's Island jail, where I worked with people diagnosed with mental illnesses, mostly of color, who had been arrested for minor substance-related and property crimes and who were struggling to develop a connection to community-based housing and treatment services. The Misdemeanor Justice Project, *Trends in Misdemeanor Arrests in New York, 1980 to 2017*, John Jay College of Criminal Justice, December 26, 2018, https://datacollaborativeforjustice.org/wp-content/uploads/2018/12/FINAL.pdf.
34. J. Wasserman, "Fear Plan Impact on Kids: See Homeless Rise," *New York Daily News*, February 10, 1995.
35. P. Donohue, "Shelter Foes Eye New Site," *New York Daily News*, February 6, 1995.
36. Office of the Mayor, Rudolph Giuliani, "Ward's Island: Manhattan Children's Psychiatric Center," 1995.
37. Office of the Mayor, "Ward's Island: Manhattan Children's Psychiatric Center."
38. S. Ferraro, "Salt in the Wounds," *New York Daily News*, January 21, 2002.
39. Odyssey House, "The George Rosenfeld Center for Recovery," March 8, 2017, https://odysseyhousenyc.org/george-rosenfeld-center-for-recovery/.
40. New York State Office of Mental Health, *Statewide Comprehensive Plan for Mental Health Services 1993–1997*, 1992; Office of the Mayor, "Randall's Island: Requests for Expressions of Interest."

41. New York State Office of Mental Health, *Statewide Comprehensive Plan*.
42. William Anthony's influential 1993 paper on recovery had a big impact on the field. W. Anthony, "Recovery from Mental Illness: The Guiding Vision of the Mental Health Service System in the 1990s," *Psychosocial Rehabilitation Journal* 16 (1993): 11–23.
43. K. Yates, M. Kunz, P. Czobor, S. Rabinowitz, J.-P. Lindenmayer, and J. Volavka, "A Cognitive, Behaviorally Based Program for Patients with Persistent Mental Illness and a History of Aggression, Crime, or Both: Structure and Correlates of Completers of the Program," *Journal of the American Academy of Psychiatry and the Law* 33 (2005): 214–22.
44. J. Parker, "No Father to His Style: The Spiritual Journey of Ol' Dirty Bastard," *Slate*, January 22, 2009, https://slate.com/culture/2009/01/the-spiritual-journey-of-ol-dirty-bastard.html.
45. E. Rems, "Wu-Tang Clan's Ol' Dirty Bastard and the Deadly Stigma of Mental Illness," *Salon*, September 24, 2019, https://www.salon.com/2019/09/24/wu-tang-clan-ol-dirty-bastard-death/.

7. "WE ARE NEW YORK'S FORGOTTEN PEOPLE": THE ISLAND NOW

1. G. B. Smith, "Woes at Wards Island Homeless Shelters Overseen by Gov. Cuomo's Sister," *City*, May 31, 2019, https://www.thecity.nyc/2019/05/31/woes-at-wards-island-homeless-shelters-overseen-by-gov-cuomo-s-sister/; B. Ostaden and D. Brand, "Troubled Wards Island Homeless Shelter Tied to Ex-Gov. Cuomo's Sister Quietly Closes," *Gothamist*, February 17, 2023, https://gothamist.com/news/troubled-wards-island-homeless-shelter-tied-to-ex-gov-cuomos-sister-quietly-closes.
2. Odyssey House, "The George Rosenfeld Center for Recovery," March 8, 2017, https://odysseyhousenyc.org/george-rosenfeld-center-for-recovery/.
3. These figures are based on an analysis of data available at NYC Planning, "2020 Census," https://www.nyc.gov/site/planning/planning-level/nyc-population/2020-census.page.
4. For references to "Ward's Island," see New York Office of Mental Health, Manhattan Psychiatric Center, https://omh.ny.gov/omhweb/facilities/mapc/internship/internship brochure.pdf; Department of Homeless Services, Keener Rapid Re-Housing Program, https://www.nyc.gov/html/hhsaccelerator/downloads/pdf/DHS%20Keener%20 Rapid%20Re-housing%20Program_2.pdf; New York City Transit, Bus Timetable: M35, https://new.mta.info/document/7606.
5. N. Oexle and P. W. Corrigan, "Understanding Mental Illness Stigma Toward Persons with Multiple Stigmatized Conditions: Implications of Intersectionality Theory," *Psychiatric Services* 69, no. 5 (2018): 587–589.
6. E. E. Toolis and P. L. Hammack, "'This Is My Community': Reproducing and Resisting Boundaries of Exclusion in Contested Public Spaces," *American Journal of Community Psychology* 56 (2015): 368–382.

7. W. T. Wright, *Out of Place: Homeless Mobilizations, Subcities, and Contested Landscapes* (Albany: State University of New York Press, 1997).
8. The study was approved by the Institutional Review Board of the City University of New York. The sample was recruited through the online research recruitment platform Prolific (https://www.prolific.com/), which verifies the legitimacy of respondents and prescreens them by country and state of residence. Three hundred participants who were confirmed as New York State residents were asked to confirm that they were New York City residents in at the point of consent to participate. Sixteen subsequently indicated that they were residents of nearby suburban areas and were therefore excluded from the analysis, leaving 284 participants. The participants were 50 percent female, 48 percent male, 1.5 percent nonbinary; 49 percent white, 23 percent Asian American, 13 percent Black, 11 percent Latino/a/x; and had a mean age of 34.5 (standard deviation = 12). Borough by borough, 31 percent resided in Brooklyn, 28 percent in Queens, 25 percent in Manhattan, 11 percent in the Bronx, and 5 percent in Staten Island. The median number of years that respondents had lived in New York City was 20 (mean = 21.5). In comparison to general New York City demographics, white, Asian American, and younger persons were overrepresented in this survey.
9. I am grateful to research assistant Francesca Bellisario for her assistance with the coding of these data.
10. C. N. Thompson, J. Baumgartner, C. Pichardo, B. Toro, L. Li, R. Arciuolo, et al., "COVID-19 Outbreak—New York City, February 29–June 1, 2020. *MMWR Morbidity and Mortality Weekly Report* 69 (2020): 1725–1729.
11. For quantitative support for this trend among the top 10 percent of earners in New York City, see E. Eisner and A. Perry, "Who Is Leaving New York State?," Fiscal Policy Institute, 2023, https://fiscalpolicy.org/wp-content/uploads/2023/12/FPI-Who-is-Leaving-Full-Report-Dec-2023.pdf. In full disclosure, I am among New York's better-off residents but remained in the city throughout the COVID-19 pandemic, though working remotely for John Jay College. I began providing in-person Assertive Community Treatment team services in July 2020, commuting by bike and meeting with clients outside, which was determined to be low-risk at that point. I did not get infected by COVID-19 until after I was vaccinated and as a result did not experience a significant course of illness. Much as I disliked remote work, I was privileged to have the opportunity to work remotely throughout the pandemic.
12. J. Tse, E. Kingman, D. LaStella, E. Chow, and S. Pearlman, "COVID-19 in a New York City Behavioral Health Housing and Treatment System," *Psychiatric Services* 72 (2021): 1209–1212; C. A. Barcella, C. Polcwiartek, G. H. Mohr, G. Hodges, K. Søndergaard, C. Niels Bang, et al., "Severe Mental Illness Is Associated with Increased Mortality and Severe Course of COVID-19," *Acta Psychiatrica Scandinavica*, 144 (2021): 82–91; M. De Hert, V. Mazereel, M. Stroobants, L. De Picker, K. Van Assche, and J. Detraux, "COVID-19-Related Mortality Risk in People with Severe Mental Illness: A Systematic and Critical Review," *Frontiers in Psychiatry* 12 (2022): 798554.

13. C. I. Aponte, A. Choi, and H. A. Duran, "COVID Tore Through NYC Homeless Shelters. But Residents Were Kept in the Dark," *The City*, June 15, 2020, https://www.thecity.nyc/2020/06/15/covid-tore-through-new-york-homeless-shelters-but-residents-were-kept-in-the-dark/.
14. D. Moses, "'People Should Never Live Like This': Life Inside a Wards Island Homeless Shelter," *AM New York/The Villager*, August 30, 2021, https://www.amny.com/news/inside-a-wards-island-homeless-shelter/. The position of public advocate is a citywide elected position; many public advocates, including recent mayor Bill DeBlasio, have gone on to be elected mayor.
15. D. Brand, "Pandemic Worsens Hard Road to Housing for Homeless New Yorkers with Health Needs," *City Limits*, September 1, 2021, https://citylimits.org/2021/09/01/pandemic-worsens-hard-road-to-housing-for-homeless-new-yorkers-with-health-needs/.
16. S. Vago and J. Fitz-Gibbon, "NYC Officials, Residents Rip Conditions at Wards Island Homeless Shelter," *New York Post*, August 30, 2021, https://nypost.com/2021/08/30/nyc-officials-residents-rip-conditions-at-wards-island-homeless-shelter/.
17. I am grateful for the assistance of a number of graduate students who helped with this project, including Sheharyar Hussain, Melissa Martinez, Samin Ali, Anna Mundy, Ashley Sedlazek, and Maria Muniz-Hernandez.
18. The project was also reviewed and approved by the CUNY Institutional Review Board.
19. J. C. Phelan, B. G. Link, and J. F. Dovidio, "Stigma and Prejudice: One Animal or Two?," *Social Science and Medicine* 67 (2008): 358–367.
20. I recruited participants by distributing an invitation through professional email lists that I belong to. I am grateful to Beatrice Quijada, Melissa Martinez, Lotus Schuller, Emma Nolasco, and Francesca Bellisario for their assistance in conducting these interviews, and to Ashley Sedlazek and Wen Ying Chen for assisting with their analysis.
21. New York State Office of Mental Health, *January 2023 Monthly Report*, 2023, https://omh.ny.gov/omhweb/transformation/docs/2023/omh-report-jan-2023.pdf.
22. Based on data from New York State Office of Mental Health, "Patient Characteristics Survey," https://omh.ny.gov/omhweb/tableau/pcs.html.
23. See Manhattan Psychiatric Center, "The Setting," https://omh.ny.gov/omhweb/facilities/mapc/internship/mpc-internship-brochure.pdf.
24. "Standard charges" for inpatient services at Manhattan Psychiatric Center as reported by the New York State Office of Mental Health, "Hospital Pricing Transparency," https://omh.ny.gov/omhweb/adults/omh-hospital-pricing-transparency.pdf. The actual cost is likely much higher. The Kaiser Family Foundation estimated that the daily cost of inpatient psychiatric services provided by state and local government was roughly $4,000 per patient/day in New York State in 2021. See Kaiser Family Foundation, "Hospital Adjusted Expenses per Inpatient Day by Ownership," https://www.kff.org/health-costs/state-indicator/expenses-per-inpatient-day-by-ownership/.

25. New York State Office of Mental Health, "Inpatient Services," https://omh.ny.gov/omhweb/facilities/mapc/inpatient_services.htm.
26. A. B. McGuire, et al., "Illness Management and Recovery: A Review of the Literature," *Psychiatric Services* 65 (2014): 171–179.
27. J. A. Lejeune, A. Northrop, and M. M. Kurtz, "A Meta-Analysis of Cognitive Remediation for Schizophrenia: Efficacy and the Role of Participant and Treatment Factors," *Schizophrenia Bulletin* 47 (2021): 997–1006.
28. J. P. Lindenmayer, S. Fregenti, G. Kang, V. Ozog, I. Ljuri, A. Khan, et al., "The Relationship of Cognitive Improvement After Cognitive Remediation with Social Functioning in Patients with Schizophrenia and Severe Cognitive Deficits," *Schizophrenia Research* 185 (2017): 154–160.
29. P. M. Grant, K. Bredemeier, and A. T. Beck, "Six-Month Follow-Up for Recovery-Oriented Cognitive Therapy for Low-Functioning Individuals with Schizophrenia," *Psychiatric Services* 68, no. 10 (2017): 997–1007.
30. New York State Office of Mental Health, "Doctoral Internship in Health Service Psychology," https://omh.ny.gov/omhweb/facilities/mapc/internship/mpc-internship-brochure.pdf.
31. P. T. Panos, J. W. Jackson, O. Hasan, and A. Panos, "Meta-Analysis and Systematic Review Assessing the Efficacy of Dialectical Behavior Therapy (DBT)," *Research on Social Work Practice* 24, no. 2 (2014): 213–223.
32. A. Venugopal, "Randall's Island Tent Shelter for Migrants Will Close at the End of February," *Gothamist*, October 9, 2024, https://gothamist.com/news/randalls-island-tent-shelter-for-migrants-will-close-at-the-end-of-february.
33. H. Meko, "What to Know About the Migrant Crisis in New York City," *New York Times*, December 6, 2023, https://www.nytimes.com/article/nyc-migrant-crisis-explained.html.
34. A. Newman, "The Latest Migrant Battleground: New York City Soccer Fields," *New York Times*, August 11, 2023, https://www.nytimes.com/2023/08/11/nyregion/nyc-migrant-crisis-eric-adams.html?searchResultPosition=3; C. Sommerfeldt, "New NYC Migrant Tent Shelter on Randalls Island Fields to House Up to 2,000, as Mayor Adams Slams Lack of Fed Help," *New York Daily News*, August 7, 2023, https://www.nydailynews.com/2023/08/07/new-nyc-migrant-tent-shelter-on-randalls-island-fields-to-house-up-to-2000-as-mayor-adams-slams-lack-of-fed-help/.
35. C. Fahy and R. Vichis, "Suing. Heckling. Cursing. N.Y.C. Protests Against Migrants Escalate," *New York Times*, September 15, 2023, https://www.nytimes.com/2023/09/15/nyregion/migrant-protests-nyc.html.
36. A. Newman, "The Latest Migrant Battleground: New York City Soccer Fields," *New York Times*, August 11, 2023, https://www.nytimes.com/2023/08/11/nyregion/nyc-migrant-crisis-eric-adams.html?searchResultPosition=3.
37. M. Kramer, "Homeless Men at Randall's Island Shelter Say City Is Treating Migrants 'Better Than Us,'" *CBS News*, October 20, 2022, https://www.cbsnews.com/newyork/news/homeless-men-at-randalls-island-shelter-criticize-city-for-treating-migrants-better-than-us/.

38. M. B. Katz, *The Undeserving Poor: America's Enduring Confrontation with Poverty* (New York: Oxford University Press, 1989).
39. D. Parra, "Outside Randall's Island Tent Shelters, Immigrants Cook to Sell or Share," *City Limits*, November 22, 2023, https://citylimits.org/2023/11/22/outside-randalls-island-tent-shelters-immigrants-cook-to-sell-or-share/.

8. THE FUTURE: WHAT CAN WARD'S ISLAND BECOME?

1. Office of the Mayor, Rudolph Giuliani, "Randall's Island Sports Foundation," 1998–2000.
2. S. Seitz and S. Miller, *The Other Islands of New York City: A History and Guide*, 3rd ed. (Woodstock VT: Countryman Press, 2011).
3. The specific wording of the question was: "There are groups that would like to convert all of the space currently being used for psychiatric and homeless services on Ward's Island into park space and to move all of those currently living on the island elsewhere. What do you think of this idea?"
4. K. Slack, "Paying for Mental Health," *New York Times*, July 14, 1993.
5. K. S. Lombardi, "County Getting Millions in Mental Health Windfall," *New York Times*, November 6, 1994.
6. New York State Office of Mental Health, "Transformation Plan," https://omh.ny.gov/omhweb/transformation/; "January 2023 Monthly Report," https://omh.ny.gov/omhweb/transformation/docs/2023/omh-report-jan-2023.pdf.
7. Center for Urban Community Services, Housing Resource Center, "Supportive Housing Options NYC: A Guide to Supportive Housing Models for Individuals Living with Mental Illness," 2016, https://www.cucs.org/wp-content/uploads/2016/11/Supportive-Housing-Options-NYC-Guide-2016.pdf.
8. J. Evelly, "Wait Times for NYCHA Apartments Doubled Last Year, as Number of Vacant Units Climb," *City Limits*, February 13, 2023, https://citylimits.org/2023/02/13/wait-times-for-nycha-apartments-doubled-last-year-as-number-of-vacant-units-climb/; NYC Continuum of Care, "New York City Supportive Housing: Client Frequently Asked Questions (FAQs), 2022, https://home.nyc.gov/assets/nycccoc/downloads/pdf/NYC%20CoC%20Supportive%20Housing%20FAQ%20for%20Clients%202022.pdf. I was unable to find an official estimate of how long the wait is for supportive housing after completion of the standard housing referral application, but the city's own support document advises that "it may take time to obtain a supportive housing unit." My own experience with helping clients apply for housing is that it can take six months to a year. After six months, a new application has to be completed because referral information is presumed to be out of date, sending the whole process back to square one. Many clients give up on the process and return to the street, stop taking medications, or resume problem substance use during this frustrating wait period.

9. Mental Health Commission of Canada, "Executive Summary from the Cross-Site At Home/Chez Soi Project," 2021, https://mentalhealthcommission.ca/resource/executive-summary-from-the-cross-site-at-home-chez-soi-project/; "National At Home/Chez Soi Final Report," 2014, https://homelesshub.ca/resource/national-home-chez-soi-final-report. In full disclosure, I have been involved in research with investigators from Pathways to Housing, which pioneered the Housing First model. However, I had no involvement in the At Home/Chez Soi study.
10. P. T. Yanos, A. Stefancic, M. J. Alexander, L. Gonzales, and B. Harney, "Association Between Housing, Personal Capacity Factors and Community Participation Among Persons with Psychiatric Disabilities," *Psychiatry Research* 260 (2018): 300–306. Probing a little further into the details of the study's findings, community participation among people living in independent scatter-site housing was better when residents had more independent living skill, whereas participation was better in congregate supportive housing for those with less independent living skill.
11. J. Foot, *The Man Who Closed the Asylums: Franco Basaglia and the Revolution in Mental Health Care* (London: Verso, 2015).
12. T. Burns and J. Foot, eds., *Basaglia's International Legacy: From Asylum to Community* (Oxford: Oxford University Press, 2020).
13. Mark Levine, Manhattan Borough President, "Breaking the Cycle: A Plan to Address NYC's Behavioral Health Crisis," 2023, https://www.manhattanbp.nyc.gov/initiatives/breaking-the-cycle/?mc_cid=8b132eb41a&mc_eid=58322675fe. This proposal also calls for the expansion of community-based services and peer support in a manner that is consistent with more reform-oriented approaches. However, the increase in inpatient beds is the component of the proposal that has received the most media attention, with the *New York Times* article featuring a picture of Manhattan Psychiatric Center.
14. Office of the Mayor, Rudolph Giuliani, "Randall's Island: Requests for Expressions of Interest," 1999.
15. See New York State Division of the Budget, "Mental Health, Office of," https://www.budget.ny.gov/pubs/archive/fy23/ex/agencies/appropdata/MentalHealthOfficeof.html.
16. See New York State Office of Mental Health, "Medicaid Reimbursement Rates," https://omh.ny.gov/omhweb/medicaid_reimbursement/; J. Tsai, G. R. Bond, and K. E. Davis, "Housing Preferences Among Adults with Dual Diagnoses in Different Stages of Treatment and Housing Types," *American Journal of Psychiatric Rehabilitation* 13, no. 4 (2010): 258–275; A. F. Lehman, S. Possidente, and F. Hawker, "The Quality of Life of Chronic Patients in a State Hospital and in Community Residences," *Psychiatric Services* 37, no. 9 (1986): 901–907.
17. J. Coltin, "Advocates: Don't Make Changes to the State's New Bail Law," *City and State, New York*, January 8, 2020, https://www.cityandstateny.com/policy/2020/01/advocates-dont-make-changes-to-the-states-new-bail-law/176550/.
18. I, along with other advocates, have criticized these statements, which cast mental illness as the cause of hate crimes, essentially scapegoating to distract from the impact

of statements from influential leaders who incite violence. See P. Yanos, "Hate Is Not a Symptom of Mental Illness," *Psychology Today*, November 18, 2018, https://www.psychologytoday.com/us/blog/written/201811/hate-is-not-symptom-mental-illness; "Monster or Human?," *Psychology Today*, August 22, 2019, https://www.psychologytoday.com/us/blog/written/201908/monster-or-human; L. Gonzalez, "Letter to the Editor: Regarding the Coverage of Mental Illness in the *New York Times*," *Medium*, April 26, 2021, https://medium.com/@lgonzales-11502/letter-to-the-editor-regarding-the-coverage-of-mental-illness-in-the-new-york-times-b5a390c2b4f5.

19. Editorial Board, "The Crazy Talk About Bringing Back Asylums," *New York Times*, June 2, 2018, https://www.nytimes.com/2018/06/02/opinion/trump-asylum-mental-health-guns.html; A. J. Harris and J. Ransom, "Behind 94 Acts of Shocking Violence, Years of Glaring Mistakes," *New York Times*, November 20, 2023, https://www.nytimes.com/2023/11/20/nyregion/nyc-mental-illness-breakdowns.html.

20. J. Ransom and A. J. Harris, "A New Push to Improve Mental Health Care for Homeless New Yorkers," *New York Times*, December 19, 2023, https://www.nytimes.com/2023/12/19/nyregion/nyc-homeless-mental-ill-violence.html?searchResultPosition=3.

21. D. Roche, "Andrew Yang Expands on Mental Illness Comments After Backlash," *Newsweek*, June 17, 2021, https://www.newsweek.com/andrew-yang-new-york-mayor-mental-illness-comments-backlash-1601443.

22. NBC News New York, "Vigil for Times Square Shove Victim Michelle Go," January 18, 2022, https://www.youtube.com/watch?v=f-tfxyWE8tw.

23. A. S. Weinstein and M. Cohen, "Young Chronic Patients and Changes in the State Hospital Population," *Hospital and Community Psychiatry* 35 (1984): 595–600.

24. A. B. Pescosolido, B. Manago, and J. Monahan, "Evolving Public Views on the Likelihood of Violence from People with Mental Illness: Stigma and Its Consequences," *Health Affairs* 38 (2019): 1735–1743.

25. B. A. Pescosolido, T. R. Medina, J. K. Martin, and J. S. Long, "The 'Backbone' of Stigma: Identifying the Global Core of Public Prejudice Associated with Mental Illness," *American Journal of Public Health* 103 (2013): 853–860.

26. The association is complex, but essentially operates like this: People exposed to negative stereotypes through the socialization process learn that serious mental illness is something that is shameful and means that one needs to live in an institution or otherwise be unable to live a satisfying life. When these individuals begin to experience psychosis or other symptoms related to serious mental illness, they avoid seeking help for fear that it will lead them to be labeled and therefore ostracized. As a participant in a recent study that I conducted stated regarding why they avoided seeking services after experiencing psychosis: "I was worried about being completely disconnected from everyone around me. . . . Would I have to live in an institution for the rest of my life, would I be able to be independent? So there were all these things going through my head." This process makes it more likely that services will not be offered until things have reached some sort of "crisis." B. C. Yu, F. H. Chio, K. K. Chan,

W. W. Mak, G. Zhang, D. Vogel, and M. H. Lai, "Associations Between Public and Self-Stigma of Help-Seeking with Help-Seeking Attitudes and Intention: A Meta-Analytic Structural Equation Modeling Approach," *Journal of Counseling Psychology* 70 no. 1 (2023): 90; S. Hussain, P. T. Yanos, C. N. Wiesepape, D. R. Samost, E. J. Myers, M. R. Munson, et al., "The Experience of Stigma and Treatment-Seeking Among Youth and Family Members Receiving First Episode Psychosis Services," *Stigma and Health*, advance online publication, 2024, https://doi.org/10.1037/sah0000507.

27. F. E. Markowitz and J. Syverson, "Race, Gender, and Homelessness Stigma: Effects of Perceived Blameworthiness and Dangerousness," *Deviance* 42 (2021): 919–931; N. L. Snow-Hill, R. N. Reeb, and J. S. Bell, "The Stigma of Homelessness as a Function of Mental Illness Comorbidity," *Stigma and Health*, March 28, 2024.
28. N. J. Kim, J. Lin, C. Hiller, C. Hildebrand, and C. Auerswald, "Analyzing U.S. Tweets for Stigma Against People Experiencing Homelessness," *Stigma and Health* 8 (2023): 187–195.
29. P. T. Yanos, J. S. DeLuca, and L. Gonzales, "The United States Has a National Prostigma Campaign: It Needs a National, Evidence-Based Antistigma Campaign to Counter It," *Stigma and Health* 5 (2020): 497–498.
30. S. Eide, "In Defense of Stigma," *National Affairs*, 2020, https://nationalaffairs.com/publications/detail/in-defense-of-stigma.
31. L. Andre, *Doctors of Deception: What They Don't Want You to Know About Shock Treatment* (New Brunswick, NJ: Rutgers University Press, 2009).
32. L. Harris, "Remembrances of Linda Andre, Leader in the Fight Against ECT," *Mad in America*, September 28, 2023, https://www.madinamerica.com/2023/09/remembrances-of-linda-andre-leader-in-the-fight-against-ect/.
33. I am grateful for the guidance of my older son, Theo, who is pursuing graduate studies in urban planning and directed me toward some helpful resources.
34. Former staff members were asked: "An alternative idea would be for permanent residences to be created on the island, for current residents as well as others, along with some amenities such as a grocery store and diner that would allow them to live more independently on the island. What do you think of this idea?" Responses included the following:

    "I love that idea. . . . And I think if they were able to absorb the patients who are already on the Island and add livable amenities, that would be really amazing. That could help people like you said, become more independent to make a life for themselves rather than living on this Island where they're pretty much surrounded by water and not much else on the Island. So I think that would be really awesome."

    "I think that's a good idea. Again, I think anything they do should really be for the people that are there. I think it's a unique opportunity to build new businesses with these things in mind—, you know, already in place. . . . To be able to integrate the people, I think would be a great way to do it rather than just imposing something and having it. Again, because it should, sort of be by the people, for the people, I'd say."

"That's great. That's what they need. That's what they need. That's what they need and they need some housing to where they could have some type of staff that could keep watch over them."

"Yes, if there can be a commitment and then you're talking about, of course, all of the money that would be required, so that people could live permanently on Ward's Island or similarly and have all of the necessities and the amenities that we all are entitled to and we all want, right now unless they've improved the public transportation, which I highly doubt, for all of my 20 years working there, there was one bus that went from Ward's and Randall's Island over to 125th Street. That's not the same as being able to go down the block literally or figuratively to your neighborhood grocery store, pharmacy, restaurant, and so on. So, yeah, in principle, I would advocate enthusiastically, that, as a desirable improvement for the patients and so on."

35. I am grateful to Lisa Green, chief program officer for residential services at the Bridge Inc., for speaking with me and offering her perspective on developing housing services; and to Paul Piwko, founder and codeveloper of the National Museum of Mental Health project, for speaking with me about my proposal and providing guidance on "best practices" within the mental health museum movement.
36. U.S. Department of Housing and Urban Development, "Low Income Housing Tax Credit (LIHTC) and Other Tax Credit Program Guidance," 2020, https://www.hud.gov/sites/dfiles/Housing/documents/2020mapguidedraftchpt14lihtcguidefinal.pdf.
37. G. Colburn and C. P. Aldern, *Homelessness Is a Housing Problem: How Structural Factors Explain U.S. Patterns* (Oakland: University of California Press, 2023).
38. See New York City Planning, "ZoLa: Zoning & Land Use Map," https://zola.planning.nyc.gov/l/zoning-district/R6?search=false; "Residence Districts: R6 - R6A - R6B," https://www.nyc.gov/site/planning/zoning/districts-tools/r6.page.
39. See New York State Office of Temporary and Disability Assistance, "Supplemental Nutrition Assistance Program (SNAP)," https://otda.ny.gov/programs/snap/.
40. P. Villotti, S. Zaniboni, M. Corbière, M., Guay, S., & Fraccaroli, F. (2018). "Reducing Perceived Stigma: Work Integration of People with Severe Mental Disorders in Italian Social Enterprise," *Psychiatric Rehabilitation Journal* 41, no. 2 (2018): 125.
41. See NAMI: National Alliance on Mental Health, https://naminycmetro.org/; Baltic Street wellness Solutions, https://balticstreet.org/.
42. See the National Museum of Mental Health Project, https://www.nmmhproject.org/. In full disclosure, I am a member of the advisory board.
43. P. Piwko, A. Orlandi, R. Folzenlogen, P. Szto, C. Yocca, R. Terrill, and P. T. Yanos, "Exhibitions About Mental Health: A Platform for Repairing Perceptions and Developing Literacy," *Museums & Social Issues* 15, nos. 1–2 (2021): 113–129.
44. In my conversation with Dr. Piwko, he praised the proposal for creating a museum on Ward's Island, stating "I just would say, I love the idea. . . . The idea that New York would be a natural place for a museum about mental health is, in my estimation, a slam dunk, from just a conceptual standpoint."

45. A. Sullivan, "How the NYS Office of Mental Health is Addressing and Reducing Stigma," *Behavioral Health News*, July 14, 2022, https://behavioralhealthnews.org/how-the-nys-office-of-mental-health-is-addressing-and-reducing-stigma/.
46. See Randall's Island Transit, https://randallsislandtransit.org/.
47. See Regional Plan Association, "The Triboro," https://rpa.org/work/reports/the-triboro.
48. See MTA (Metropolitan Transit Authority), "Penn Station Access," https://new.mta.info/project/penn-station-access.
49. See Citi Bike, "Bike NYC. Like, All of It," https://citibikenyc.com/.
50. V. Chakrabarti, "How to Make Room for One Million New Yorkers," *New York Times*, December 30, 2023, https://www.nytimes.com/interactive/2023/12/30/opinion/new-york-housing-solution.html; NYC Department of Planning, "City of Yes," https://www.nyc.gov/site/planning/plans/city-of-yes/city-of-yes-housing-opportunity.page.
51. A. L. Huxtable, "A Plan for Welfare Island Is Unveiled," *New York Times*, October 10, 1969.
52. E. E. Ansbury, "Welfare Is: A Problem for Housing," *New York Times*, February 16, 1972; P. Goldberger, "A Broader Horizon Is in the Offing for Roosevelt Island," *New York Times*, September 27, 1977.
53. See Wikipedia, "Roosevelt Island," last modified November 16, 2024, 7:17 (UTC), https://en.wikipedia.org/wiki/Roosevelt_Island.
54. A. Wachs, "Plan Would Surround Poughkeepsie's Long-Vacant Hudson River Psychiatric Center with Suburban Homes, Shopping," *Architect's Newspaper*, September 10, 2015, https://www.archpaper.com/2015/09/long-vacant-hudson-river-psychiatric-center-poughkeepsie-will-transformed-mixed-use-development/.
55. G. Wilson, "Hudson Heritage: Demolition at Former Psychiatric Center Lifts Veil on Mysterious Site," *Poughkeepsie Journal*, July 31, 2019, https://www.poughkeepsiejournal.com/story/news/local/2019/07/31/hudson-heritage-project-transform-hudson-river-psychiatric-center/1639202001/.
56. J. Braithwaite, "The Fundamentals of Restorative Justice," in *A Kind of Mending: Restorative Justice in the Pacific Islands*, ed. S. Dinnen (Canberra: Australian National University, ANU E Press, 2003), 35–43.

INDEX

Note: page numbers in italics refer to figures.

Action for Mental Health (Joint Commission on Mental Illness and Health), 60
Adams, Eric, 140n10
Addis, Wendy, 72
African American patients at Manhattan State Hospital: diagnostic reasons for admission, 50, 145n18; documentary evidence on, 49–50
African American patients at New York City Asylum for the Insane: documentary evidence on, 29, 30–31; as likely not segregated, 30; and scientific racism theories, 29
African Americans: in asylums, typical segregation of, 30; marginalized, increased risk of psychosis in, 50; in New York State, rate of admission to mental hospitals, mid twentieth century, 49–50; and 19th-century theories on psychological stress in freed slaves, 29; and racialization of schizophrenia, 63, 145n18
alcohol and substance abuse, and homelessness, 77–78, 79
Alcoholics Anonymous: first chapter at Manhattan State Hospital, 51–52; founding of, 145n21
Aldern, Clayton Page, 76
American Psychiatric Association: commendation of Manhattan Psychiatric Center artwork, 64; origin in AMSAII, 51, 340
AMSAII. *See* Association of Medical Superintendents of American Institutions for the Insane
Andre, Linda, 127
Assertive Community Treatment, 124
Association of Medical Superintendents of American Institutions for the Insane (AMSAII), 30, 51
asylums, early: cost per patient, 24, 26, 142n25; moral treatment model, 24, 27, 50; in New York City, 24–25; origin and purpose of, 23–24. *See also* New York City Asylum for the Insane, Ward's Island branch
"Asylums for Colored Persons" (Galt), 30
At Home/Chez Soi study, 122

automobile age, and remote asylum locations, 44

Baltic Street AEH, 132
Basaglia, Franco, 122–123
Benepe, Adrian, 95
Bicetre Hospital (Paris), 15, 24
Blackwell Island (Roosevelt Island): author's family's residence on, 136; as former asylum site, 14, 135; Homeopathic Hospital move to, 22; other city institutions on, 25; redevelopment of, 135–136
Blackwell Island asylum: Bly's exposé of conditions in, 33–34; as first New York City public asylum, 24; poor conditions in, 25; switch to all-women's facility, 25
Bloomberg, Michael, 93
Bloomingdale Asylum, 24, 142n17, 142n19
Bly, Nelly (Elizabeth Jane Cochrane), 33–34
Boden, Aimee, 88, 92, 152n9
Buckley School, 88
bus line to Ward's Island (M35): and exposure of patients to outside influences, 62–63; Harlem terminus of, as street drug market, 13, 63, 136–137; as infrequent and unreliable, 5, 13, 106, 144n11; introduction of, 45–46; mix of homeless people and children on, 74; need for expanded or alternative services, 133–134; as residents' only access to stores and services, 106–107, 109, 131

Callahan, Robert, 74–75
Callahan Consent Decree, 74–75
Charpentier, Paul, 57
chlorpromazine (Thorazine): and deinstitutionalization movement, 58, 60; introduction of, 56–57
City Advisory Commission on Care of the Insane, 34
Clarke Thomas Men's Shelter, 97; current number of residents, 102; founding of, 97; residents' lack of vibrancy, 116; residents' objections to new migrant tent shelter, 115–116
Coalition for the Homeless, 72, 78, 96
Cochrane, Elizabeth Jane (Nelly Bly), 33–34
cognitive behavior therapy, 11, 112
cognitive frame theory, and neighborhood rebranding, 91
cognitive remediation therapy, 112
Cohen, Karen, 88, 91–92, 93, 119
Colburn, Gregg, 76
community-based care, introduction of, 59–60
community-based housing and services: as cheaper and more successful than inpatient treatment, 124; cost of, 124
Community Mental Health Reinvestment Act (New York State, 1993), 121
Community Mental Health Services Act (New York State, 1954), 59
Community Mental Health Services Act (US, 1963), 65
contested spaces in gentrifying cities, 103–104
COVID-19 pandemic: impact on New York City, 105–106; and public attention to Ward's Island homeless shelters, 106–107; and shelter residents' risk factors, 106
crack cocaine, and demoralization of 1990s, 87
criminal justice system, people with mental illness in: "not competent to stand trial" status, 81–82; not guilty by reason of insanity (NGRI) status, 81–82; treatment of most within system, 81–82
Crownsville Asylum (Maryland), 30

Damnation Island (Horn), 25
deinstitutionalization movement: in 1950s, 58; community-based care introduction, 59–60; community support for, 58; and decline in population at Manhattan

Psychiatric Center, 65; emergence of, 36, 45; and parole/convalescent care, 58; public support for, 60
DeLuca, Joseph, 140n19
Democratic Party figures: calls for removal of people with mental illness from public spaces, 124, 125; and negative stereotypes of homeless persons, 126–127
Denber, Herman, 58–59, 60
Densen-Gerber, Judianne, 68
Deutsch, Albert, 60
Dewey, John, 54
dialectical behavior therapy (DBT) at Manhattan Psychiatric Center, 112
Dickens, Charles, 25
Dinkins, David, 88
Downs, Hugh, 58
drug abuse: and 1990s' demoralization in New York City, 87; higher rate in whites vs. people of color, 151n3
DSM-II, and racialization of schizophrenia, 63
Dunlap Building, opening of, 57

Echeverria, M. G., 25, 31
Economic Development Corporation of New York City, 92
Eide, Stephen, 126
Eisenhower, Dwight D., 54, 60
elderly patients: development of nursing homes for, 65; inappropriate dumping at Manhattan State Hospital, 32, 48–49, 56
Ellis Island, opening of, 20
Emigrant Refuge and Hospital, 20–21, *21*, 33
English, T. J., 62
eugenics movement: and anti-immigrant sentiment in 19th-century U.S., 28–29; and psychiatric research, 49

footbridge to Ward's Island. *See* Ward's Island footbridge from East Harlem
Foucault, Michele, 15
French Connection, The (film), 68–69, *69*

future of Ward's Island. *See* proposal for Ward's Island future; Ward's Island future with expanded Manhattan Psychiatric Center (future version 2); Ward's Island future without psychiatric hospitals (future version 1)

Galt, John M., 30
Genovese, Kitty, 61–62
gentrification: and contested spaces, 103–104; and displacement of lower-income residents, 91; and increased park space, 91
gentrification in New York City: Bloomberg and, 93; and loss of affordable housing stock, 75–76, 79; and neighborhood rebranding, 89–91; and Ward Island development as park, 120
George Rosenfeld Center for Recovery. *See* Odyssey House (Ward's Island)
Giuliani, Rudy, 92, 96, 97, 153n33
Gotbaum, Betsy, 88
Grob, Gerald, 60

Harlem Valley State Hospital, 47, 48, 121
Hayes, Robert, 72, 73
Hell Gate Bridge, 39; construction of, 38–39; in *The French Connection*, 68–69, *69*; and future subway line to Ward's Island, 133–134; and Ward's Island access, 39, 144n1
Hellgate channel, 18–19
HELP USA shelter, 97, 102
Heyman, Marcus, 35
HIV epidemic in New York City, 87, 151n4
homelessness: as national crisis, 80; overrepresentation of Black and Hispanic persons, 80; overrepresentation of people with mental illness, 80–81; state hospitalization as cause of, 127

homelessness, stigmatization of: increase of, when combined with mental illness or being Black, 126; pro-stigma campaigns, 126–127; and public fear, 126; and public's view of hospitalization as cure for homelessness, 127; stigma reduction features in author's proposal for Ward's Island redevelopment, 132, 133, 135

homelessness in New York City: alcohol and substance abuse and, 77–78, 79; and attacks on homeless by local youths, 85; causes of, 75–81; city-state cooperation in building housing for people with mental illness, 80, 96; and constitutional right to shelter, 72; decline in affordable housing stock and, 75–76, 79; deinstitutionalization movement and, 78, 79; disputes between city vs. state over, 75–76, 80; fluctuation of shelter population in 1990s, 95; high arrest rates of homeless, 96, 153n33; increase in 1970s–80s, 71–72; landlord abandonments and, 76; late 1970s' changing demographic of, 72; psychiatric problems among homeless, 72, 77; shelters, history of, 71–72; shorter stays at state psychiatric hospitals and, 78; and single-room occupancy hotels, tax incentives to close, 75–76; tightening of admission criteria at state hospitals and, 76–77, 78; War on Drugs and, 79–80; young adult chronic psychiatric patients and, 77–78, 79

homeless shelters on Ward's Island: and COVID-19 vulnerability of residents, 106; current number of residents, 102; public attention to, in COVID-19 pandemic, 106–107; residents' complaints about, 106–107; residents' objections to new migrant tent shelter, 115–116. See also Clarke Thomas Men's Shelter; HELP USA shelter; Jewish Board community residence; Keener Men's Shelter

Homeopathic Hospital on Ward's Island, 22
Hopper, Kim, 71, 72, 76, 78
Horn, Stacy, 25
housing: construction of, in author's proposal for Ward's Island future, 129–130; as issue for discharged mental patients, 78; patients' loss of, during residence in state psychiatric hospitals, 2, 12. See also community-based housing and services
Housing First model: author's proposal for Ward's Island future and, 129; cost of, 122, 124; potential benefits to deinstitutionalized patients, 121–122, 158n8; and scatter-site vs. congregate supportive housing, 121, 122, 159n10
Hudson River Psychiatric Center, 136

Icahn Stadium, 5, 93
immigrants: anti-immigrant sentiment in U.S. and, 28–29, 118–119; and immigration as risk factor for schizophrenia, 28; insane, deportation of, 27; as majority of population in Manhattan State Hospital, 49, 118; as majority of population of New York City Asylum for the Insane, 27–28, 33; State Emigrant Refuge and Hospital on Ward's Island (19th century), 14, 20–21, 21, 34, 118. See also migrant tent shelter on Ward's Island
Impellitteri, Vincent, 55
Inebriate Asylum on Ward's Island, 14, 22, 23, 33
institutionalization of homeless people, increasing public support for, 127
institutionalization of people with mental illness: and false association of mental illness with violence, 124, 159–160n18; increasing public support for, 123, 124–125
isolation of institutions for people with mental illness: automobile age and, 44;

closing of Ward's Island facilities and, 120; East River islands as well-suited for, 24; functions served by, 15; history of, 15–16; New York City Asylum for the Insane and, 26; and "not in my backyard" (NIMBY) mentality, 15, 140–141n20; and problems of staffing and provisioning, 25, 26; and terror management theory, 140n19; views of Ward's Island employees on, 110

isolation of marginalized people: functions served by, 15; as purpose of Ward's Island institutions, 16, 67, 103, 106–107, 118, 120, 137

Italy: closing of state psychiatric hospitals (Trieste Model), 122–123; and "social enterprise" model, 131–132, 137

James, Letitia, 125
Jewish Board community residence, 102, 108, 135
Jewish Board for Family and Children's Services, 102
Joint Commission on Mental Illness and Health, 60
Jones, Russell (aka Ol' Dirty Bastard), 99–100, 132
Joplin, Scott, 29, 132

Keener Building, 67; housing of children with severe intellectual disabilities in 1970s, 66–67; repurposing as homeless shelter, 72–73
Keener Men's Shelter: current number of residents, 102; expansion of, 73–74, 81; fatal attack on residents by local youths, 84–86; impact on Ward's Island residents, 149n10; opening of, 72–73, 74; opposition to, 73, 74; proposal for repurposing as museum, 132; residents' lack of vibrancy, 116; standards required by Callahan Consent Decree, 74–75

"keeping people away." *See* isolation of institutions for people with mental illness; isolation of marginalized people
Kellogg, Theodore H., 25
Kirby Building: conversion to Kirby Forensic Psychiatric Center, 81; opening of, 58; proposal for future of, 129
Kirby Forensic Psychiatric Center: cost per patient, 111; current number of residents, 102, 111; opening of, 81–82; patient demographics, 82, 111; potential closing, staff's opinions on, 119–121; proposal for future of, 128–129; recent employees' views on, 109–110; security at, 82, 83; staff views on treatment quality, 112–113; types of patients in, 81–82, 111
Koch, Edward, 71, 72–73, 74, 78
Koz, Gabriel, 64–66, 73, 82–84, 112, 151n4
Kraepelin, Emil, 37

Laborit, Henri, 57
La Guardia, Fiorello, 43
Legal Aid Society, 72, 73
Lehner, Theresa, 35
Levine, Mark, 123, 124
Levitt, Arthur, 64
Lindenmayer, J. P., 112

Mabon, William, 35, 67
MacCurdy, Frederick, 54
MacDonald, Alexander: and accommodations for non-Protestant Asylum patients, 28; discharge of patients determined not to be insane, 31–32; and investigations of New York City Asylum, 34; reports on conditions at asylum, 26–28, 31, 34; and state takeover of New York City Asylum, 34–35; as superintendent of New York City Asylum for the Insane, 25–26
Mad Among Us, The (Grob), 60
Madness and Civilization (Foucault), 15

Madness in the City of Magnificent Intentions (Summers), 29

Malzberg, Benjamin, 33, 49–50, 145n18

Manhattan Children's Psychiatric Center (MCPC): closing of, 96; construction of, 66; opposition to homeless shelter on Ward Island, 73, 74; population served, 66, 96–97; reuse of building for Clarke Thomas Men's Shelter, 97; types of treatment, 66

Manhattan Psychiatric Center, 4; author's father as psychiatrist at, 3; author's visits to patient in, 2–3, 6, 8–13; author's work as volunteer in, 6–8, 84; blocked access to Ward's Island recreation facilities, 6, 11, 13; budget reductions of early 1980s, 83; calls for funding and staff increases, 65; cost per patient, 65–66, 111, 156n24; current number of residents, 102, 110; current treatment methods, 111–112; decline in population in 1990s, 98; decline in quality of care in 1980s, 83–84; and deinstitutionalization movement, 65, 78; fluctuation of population over its history, 110; and HELP USA shelter, 102; as high-security environment, 8; and housing for discharged patients, 78; increase in special needs patients in 1990s, 98–99; Jewish Board community residence, 102, 108, 135; lengthy approval process for release from, 12; Manhattan State Hospital's renaming as, 64; number of patients, 3; as oldest institution on Ward's Island, 110; opposition to homeless shelter on Ward Island, 73; patient beaten to death by aides in 1980s, 83; patient demographics in 1990s, 99; patient demographics today, 111; potential closing, and benefits to residents of Housing First alternatives, 121–122, 158n8; potential closing, staff's opinions on, 119–121; proposal for future of, 128–129; and psychiatric rehabilitation movement, 99; psychiatrists' deaths from AIDS, 151n4; recent employees' views on, 109–110; reduced capacity in 1980s, 64; Russell Jones (aka Ol' Dirty Bastard) as patient at, 99–100, 132; sculpture garden and indoor art added to, 64; staff views on treatment quality, 112–113; and STAIR, 99; themes in history of, 16–17; Transitional Living Residence, 102, 127; types of patients and length of stay, 110–111; as unique concentration of institutions, 16. *See also* Manhattan State Hospital; New York City Asylum for the Insane, Ward's Island branch; Ward's Island

Manhattan State Hospital: Black patients, documentary evidence of, 49–50; budget cuts of 1970s, 63–64, 147n24; building of staff housing, 35; chronic overcrowding in, 37; community-based care, introduction of, 59–60; concerns about land ceded for Wastewater Treatment Plant, 40, 41; crime problems after opening of Ward's Island Park, 61–62; deadly fire (1923), 36, 144n1; decision to save and rebuild, 52–53, 54; and deinstitutionalization movement, 36, 45, 58; deterioration in 1970s, factors in, 60–64; deterioration of buildings in expectation of closure, 53; development of medical approach to treatment, 36–37; golden years of 1957-1961, 57; high percentage of immigrants in, 49; inappropriate dumping of elderly and decrepit individuals at, 48–49, 56; infrastructure improvements, 36; Keener Building repurposed as facility for children with severe intellectual disabilities, 66–67, 67; MacDonald's period as superintendent, 35; new high-rise buildings, opening of, 54, 57, 58; "open hospital" experiment, 57–59,

62–63; planned removal in Ward's Island Park plan, 43–44; poor conditions in, 35–36, 143n47; proximity to street drug markets, 63; renaming as Manhattan Psychiatric Center, 64; repurposing of Mabon Building for Odyssey House, 67–68, 98; research unit, 58–59; state comptroller's report condemning, 64; as successor to New York City Asylum, 34–35; superintendents, 35; transfer of patients into, in 1970s, 64; transfer of patients to other state hospitals, before planned closing, 35, 43–45, 47–48; types of treatments in, 37, 50–51, 56–57, 58, 59
marginalized people: functions served by isolation of, 15; increased risk of psychosis in, 50; isolation of, as purpose of Ward's Island institutions, 16, 118, 120, 137
Martinez, Pablo, 83
MCPC. *See* Manhattan Children's Psychiatric Center
media, and negative stereotypes of homeless persons, 126
"Mental Health: Mind Matters" traveling exhibit, 133
mental health museum for Ward's Island: author's proposal for, 132–133, 162n44; in Moses' early plan for Island redevelopment, 46
mental illness, stigmatization of: false association with violence, 124, 159–160n18; public support for removal from public spaces, 123, 124–127, 159–160n18; stigma reduction features in author's proposal for Ward's Island redevelopment, 132, 133, 135. *See also* institutionalization of people with mental illness; isolation of institutions for people with mental illness
Metropolitan Hospital, 22
Metropolitan Transit Authority (MTA), 134
Metzl, Jonathan, 63, 145n18

Meyer, Adolf, 36–37, 51
Meyer Building: opening of, 58; patients' escape from, 82
microaggressions, of park advocates against Ward's Island's institutional residents, 92
migrant tent shelter on Ward's Island, 13, 113–117, *114*; city officials' description of location as Randall's Island, 114, 116; future of, as unclear, 135; homeless shelters residents' criticisms of, 115–116; lack of neighborhood to object to, 114–115; origin of migrants in, 114, 118; plans to close, 114; vibrant life at, 116, *116*
moral treatment model, 24, 27, 50
Moses, Robert: and La Guardia administration, 43; on Manhattan State Hospital closing, 48; power over city planning, 41–43; and Triborough Bridge, 43, 45; and Ward's Island footbridge, 55–56; and Ward's Island Park plan, 43, 44–45, 53, 54, 101
Moynihan, Daniel Patrick, 62

National Alliance on Mental Illness–New York City chapter, 132
National Museum of Mental Health Project, 132
National Rifle Association, 126
Nazi Germany, and eugenics, 49
neighborhood rebranding, urban gentrification and, 89–91
Nelly Bly (Elizabeth Jane Cochrane), 33–34
New Deal, and Triborough Bridge construction, 43
New York City: "City of Yes" proposal, 135; COVID-19 pandemic and, 105–106; criteria for detaining people on mental health grounds, 140n10; and "de-civilizing" process of 1960s, 61; fall of crime rates under Giuliani, 92; high crime rates in 1960s–70s, 61–62; rise in drug abuse in 1960s, 62; violence and demoralization of 1990s, 87

New York City Asylum for the Insane, Ward's Island branch: abysmal conditions in, 25–26; accommodations for non-Protestant patients, 28; activities for patients, 26–27; architectural style of, 26, 27; chronic overcrowding in, 33; cost per patient, 26; dumping of old and decrepit individuals on, 32; establishment as all-male facility, 25; expansion of, 33; growth in patient population, 32, 32–33; high percentage of immigrants in, 27–28; investigations leading to reforms at, 34; MacDonald's tenure as superintendent, 25–28, 31–32, 34; mistreatment of patients, 31; and moral treatment model, 27; moving of Blackwell Islands' female patients to, 34; multiple languages of immigrant patients as obstacle, 28; *New York Herald* exposé on conditions in, 34; patients as mostly immigrants, 33; patient-to-staff ratios, 31; poorly paid and unqualified staff, 31; as predecessor of Manhattan Psychiatric Center, 14, 23; recruiting of staff from city jail, 31; superintendents of, 25, 31; superintendents' reports on poor conditions in, 26; turn-over to state control, 34–35; wrongly-committed patients, 31–32. *See also* African American patients at New York City Asylum for the Insane

New York Herald exposé on New York City Asylum, 34

New York State Commission on Quality Care for the Mentally Disabled: Community Mental Health Reinvestment Act of 1993, 121; harsh report on Manhattan Psychiatric Center, 83–84, 99

New York State Office of Mental Health: anti-stigma campaign of, 133; author's proposal for Ward's Island and, 130; and cost of expanding Manhattan Psychiatric Center, 123; decline of, in 1980s, 83; and discharge of patients without housing, 78; reallocation of funds from closed hospitals, 121; and sale of land from former hospitals, 136; state hospitals as small segment of facilities licensed by, 76–77, 111

New York state psychiatric hospitals, sharp reduction in patients, 1955–1980, 65

New York Times: and false association of mental illness with violence, 124; and negative stereotypes of homeless persons, 126–27

1960s: "de-civilizing" process in, 61; high crime rates in, 61–62

"not competent to stand trial" patients, 81–82

not guilty by reason of insanity (NGRI) patients, 81–82

"not in my backyard" (NIMBY) mentality: and creation of Ward's Island institutions, 19–20, 97, 114–115; and homeless shelters, 140–141n20; and isolation of people with mental illness, 15, 140–141n20; and Manhattan Psychiatric Center location, 127; and migrant shelters, 119

Odyssey House (Ward's Island) [now George Rosenfeld Center for Recovery]: in author's plan for Ward's Island future, 135; current number of residents, 102; founding of, 67; number of patients, 98; renovations in 2010s, 98; treatment provided by, 67

Office of Mental Health. *See* New York State Office of Mental Health

Other Islands of New York City, The (Seitz and Miller), 119

parks: in author's plan for Ward's Island redevelopment, 130–131; gentrification and, 91. *See also* Randall's Island Sports Foundation/Park Alliance (RISF/RIPA);

Ward's Island Park; Ward's Island public recreation facilities
Pataki, George, 96, 121
Penney, Darby, 35
Pinel, Philippe, 24
Pinker, Steven, 61
Piwko, Paul, 132, 162n44
police: 1960s' policy of benign neglect in poor minority neighborhoods, 62; psychiatric patients' bad experiences with, 10
proposal for Ward's Island future, 127–137; addition of new park space, 131; addition of stores and essential services for island residents, 131–132; asylum seekers and, 135; Clarke Thomas shelter, demolition of, 129, 131; consistency with Housing First approach, 129; consolidation of psychiatric hospitals into one building, 128–129; construction of mixed population housing for low-income people and people with serious mental illness, 129–130; construction of subsidized housing for formerly homeless, 129; as evidence-based, 128, 129, 131–132; features for stigma reduction, 132, 133, 135; improved transportation to and on Island, 133–134; input of former staff on, 161–162n34; Keener shelter repurposing as museum, 131, 132; likely improvements to residents' lives from, 136–137; mental health museum, 132–133; Odyssey House and existing community residences and, 135; precedents for, 135–136; public library focused on mental health, 133; removal of fencing separating park and housing, 130–131; residents' preference for remaining on island and, 128; and restorative justice, 137; social justice as goal of, 127–128, 136; summary of, 134–135
psychiatric rehabilitation approach: evidence base for, 99; at Manhattan Psychiatric Center, 84, 99

psychiatry, establishment as field, 51
psychobiology, as term, 37
psychotropic drugs, and deinstitutionalization movement, 58

race: and eugenics, 28–29, 49; first mention of, in Ward's Island hospital records, 49
racial and economic divide in New York City, 10, 16
racism, structural, and psychosis, 50
Randall's Island: aerial view, 4; landfill uniting Ward's Island and, 3, 68, 89; location of, 3; plan to convert to park, 41; public recreation facilities on, 5–6, 16; public's awareness of, 105; and Triborough Bridge construction, 45
Randall's Island Park Alliance (RIPA). *See* Randall's Island Sports Foundation/Park Alliance (RISF/RIPA)
Randall's Island Sports Foundation/Park Alliance (RISF/RIPA): controversy over private school usage of fields, 94–96; fencing-off of institutions, 92; and gentrification, 91; Icahn Stadium and other large projects, 93–94; increased use of parks following renovations, 94; judges' rejection of renovation funds offered by, 95; as public-private partnership, 88–89, 152n9; and rebranding of Randall's and Ward's Islands, 89–91; rejuvenation of Ward's and Randall's Island parks and playing fields, 88–89, 92–94, 93, 101; removal of Ward's Island's institutions as ultimate goal of, 91–92, 119; renaming as Randall's Island Park Alliance (RIPA), 94; success in publicizing park facilities, 105; use of Randall's Island name for all Ward's and Randall's Island facilities, 89, 90; on Ward's Island's institutional residents as eyesores, 92
Randall's Island Transit proposal, 133
Reed, Lou, 63, 87

Regional Plan Association of New York, 41, 133–134
restorative history, 17
restorative justice, 137
RIPA. *See* Randall's Island Sports Foundation/Park Alliance (RISF/RIPA)
RISF. *See* Randall's Island Sports Foundation/Park Alliance (RISF/RIPA)
Rivera, Geraldo, 67
Roosevelt, Franklin D., 41
Roosevelt Island. *See* Blackwell Island (Roosevelt Island)

St. Elizabeth's Asylum (Washington, DC), 30
Savage City, The (English), 62
Service for Treatment and Abatement of Interpersonal Risk (STAIR), 99
Shame of the States, The (Deutsch), 60
Siegel, Norman, 94
Smith, Al, 36
social enterprise model, 131–132, 137
SSI. *See* supplemental security income
STAIR (Service for Treatment and Abatement of Interpersonal Risk), 99
Stastny, Peter, 35
State Emigrant Refuge and Hospital on Ward's Island (nineteenth century), 14, 20–21, *21*, 34
state psychiatric hospitals: advocates for closure of, 122–123; destructive effects of long stays in, 2, 12; in New York City, 3, 139n4; potential reallocation of funds for community-based programs, 121; sharp reduction in patients, 1955–1980, 65
stigma theory, 15
stigmatization. *See* homelessness, stigmatization of; mental illness, stigmatization of
Summers, Martin, 29
supplemental security income (SSI): discontinuation during residence in state psychiatric hospitals, 2; and need for subsidized housing for homeless, 129; and New York City rents, 76
syphilis, psychosis from: decline in admissions due to, 144–145n15; and institutionalization, 24, 29, 33

Ten Days in a Madhouse (Bly), 33–34
terror management theory, 140n19
transitional living residences (TLRs), discharging of patients to, 12, 45, 78, 102, 108, 127
Travis, John, 48–49, 58
treatment malls in Manhattan Psychiatric Center, 111–112, 113
treatment of mental illness: antipsychotic medications, introduction of, 56–57, 58; antipsychotic medications, over-reliance on, 84; and chlorpromazine (Thorazine), 56–57; cognitive behavior therapy, 112; cognitive remediation therapy, 112; community-based care, introduction of, 59–60; dialectical behavior therapy (DBT), 112; early medications, 50; early psychosocial treatments, 51–52; early psychosurgery techniques, 51, 58; electric shock therapy, 50; hydrotherapy, 37, 50, 51; insulin shock therapy, 50, 58; at Manhattan Psychiatric Center, 111–112; at Manhattan State Hospital, 37, 50–51, 56–57, 58, 59; medical approach, development of, 36–37, 50–51, 56–57; moral treatment model in early asylums, 24, 27, 50; occupational therapy, 28, 37, 50, 51; psychiatric rehabilitation approach, 84; psychopharmacology, 112; psychotherapy, 57–58, 59; psychotropic drug revolution and, 56–57, 58; racialization of schizophrenia, 63, 145n18; rehab therapy, 112; staff shortages and, 51; treatment malls, 111–112, 113; Wellness Self-Management programs, 111
Triborough Bridge (Robert F. Kennedy Bridge): construction of, 45; and

INDEX

improved access to Ward's Island in future, 133; and New Deal funds, 43; off-ramp to Randall's and Ward's Islands, 3, 45; pedestrian path to Randall's and Ward's Island, 5–6; and shutdown of ferry service, 45; traffic volume on, 3; and Ward's Island Park plans, 43, 45

Trieste Model of psychiatric services, 123

Tyler, Andrew, 72

Ward, Jasper and Bartholomew, 19

Ward's Island: access improvements, proposals for, 133–134; access to, 3–6, 13, 14, 45–46, 144n11; aerial view of, 4; author's childhood on, 2–3, 6, 7, 9, 39, 69–70, 70; and contested spaces in gentrifying cities, 103–104; lack of services and amenities, 13, 36; landfill uniting Randall's Island and, 3, 68, 89; limiting of name to institutional locations only, 89, 97–98, 101, 102–103; location of, 3; New Yorkers' limited awareness of, 3, 101, 104–105, 139–140n8, 155n8; ongoing isolation of patients on, 106–107; polarization between parks for privileged and institutions for marginalized, 100, 101, 102–103, 103, 118; polarization, employees' views on, 109–110; polarization, resident's views on, 108–109; population, in 2010 and 2020, 102; residents' lack of access to public recreation facilities, 6, 11, 13

Ward's Island, history of: access to, in nineteenth century, 19, 20, 38; author's identity and, 17; city Wastewater Treatment Plant construction, 40, 40, 41; colonial period and American Revolution, 18–19, 141n1; cotton factory, 19; first public institutions, 19–22, 21, 23; graveyard for indigents (potter's field), 14, 21–22; Hell Gate Bridge construction, 38–39, 39; Island's early names, 18; isolation, problems caused by, 25, 26, 38;

map of (1860s), 23, 141–142n12; purchase and development by Ward brothers, 19; purchase by City, 19–20, 22; themes in, 16–17; and War of 1812, 19. *See also* Ward's Island Park

Ward's Island footbridge from East Harlem: construction of, 55, 55–56; and crime problems on Ward's Island, 61–62, 85, 86; and local youths' attack on Keener Shelter residents, 85–86; poor access to, 56; renaming as 103rd Street Footbridge, 94; reopening of, after RISF park renovations, 94

Ward's Island future with expanded Manhattan Psychiatric Center (future, version 2), 123–127; community-based housing and, 124; cost of, 123; and expansion of community-based services, 159n13; and public support for removal of homeless people with mental illness, 123, 124–127, 159–160n18; and treatment avoidance, 126, 160–161n26

Ward's Island future without psychiatric hospitals (future, version 1), 119–123; potential benefits of Housing First alternatives, 121–122, 158n8; staff's opinions on, 119–121; as type of gentrification, 120

Ward's Island institutional facilities, 5, 13; current facilities, 101–102; as "dumping ground" for marginalized people, 16, 67, 103, 106–107, 118, 120, 137; first nineteenth-century institutions, 19–22, 21, 23; history of, 14; new facilities added in 1970s, 66–68; removal of, as RISF goal, 91–92. *See also* Clarke Thomas Men's Shelter; HELP USA shelter; Inebriate Asylum on Ward's Island; Jewish Board community residence; Keener Men's Shelter; Kirby Forensic Psychiatric Center; Manhattan Children's Psychiatric Center; Manhattan Psychiatric Center; Manhattan State

Ward's Island institutional facilities (*continued*)
Hospital; migrant tent shelter on Ward's Island; New York City Asylum for the Insane, Ward's Island branch; Odyssey House (Ward's Island)

Ward's Island Park, 41–46, *46*; amount of available land and, 41, *42*; author's childhood memories of, 69–70; compromise plan leaving Manhattan State Hospital in place, 52–53, 54; funding of, 43; Moses's plan for, 43, 44–45, 53, 54, 101; and pedestrian bridge, 46; period of high crime and low public use, 68–69, 85–86; planned health museum, 46; plan to remove all structures, 44; problems of public access, 68; supporters of plan for, 41–43; Triborough Bridge and, 43, 45

Ward's Island public recreation facilities, 6, 8, *10*; development of, 54–55; facilities, in 1950s, 55; and fear of State Hospital, 56; private schools' takeover and restoration of, 88; residents' lack of access to, 6, *11*, 13, 108–109; as underused, due to access problems, 56. *See also* Randall's Island Sports Foundation (RISF); Ward's Island Park

Ward's Island residents: author's interviews of, 107–109; intersecting stigmatized identities of, 103; isolation of, 13; as mostly Black and Latino/a/x marginalized people, 13, 16, 118; number of, 13; on positive aspects of Island, 109; as predominantly people of color, 102, 103; on their stigmatized identity and isolation, 108–109

War on Drugs: disproportionate effect on people of color, 79, 80; and homelessness, 79–80; and people with serious mental illness in prisons, 94

Washington Heights, efforts to rebrand, 91

Washington Square Park, 22

Wastewater Treatment Plant on Ward's Island: construction of, 40, *40*, 41; as invisible to most New Yorkers, 101

Wellness Self-Management program at Manhattan Psychiatric Center, 111

Williams, Jumaane, 106, 107

Willowbrook State School, 67

World War II, and need for Manhattan State Hospital services, 52–53

Wright, Talmadge, 103–104

Yang, Andrew, 125

GPSR Authorized Representative: Easy Access System Europe, Mustamäe tee
50, 10621 Tallinn, Estonia, gpsr.requests@easproject.com